A LIFE.
A FINGER.
A PEA UP
A NOSE.

A LIFE.
A FINGER.
A PEA UP
A NOSE.

BABY AND CHILD FIRST AID

SARAH HUNSTEAD RN (BNurs) MN

HarperCollins*Publishers*

HarperCollins*Publishers*

First published in Australia in 2013 by CPR Kids Pty Ltd
This revised edition published in 2017
by HarperCollins*Publishers* Australia Pty Limited
ABN 36 009 913 517
harpercollins.com.au

HarperCollins*Publishers*
Level 13, 201 Elizabeth Street, Sydney NSW 2000, Australia
Unit D1, 63 Apollo Drive, Rosedale, Auckland 0632, New Zealand
A 53, Sector 57, Noida, UP, India
1 London Bridge Street, London, SE1 9GF, United Kingdom
2 Bloor Street East, 20th floor, Toronto, Ontario M4W 1A8, Canada
195 Broadway, New York NY 10007, USA

ISBN 9781460753248 (pbk)
ISBN 9781460707876 (e-book)

Cover image by Lauren Burke/Getty Images
Cover design by Hazel Lam, HarperCollins Design Studio
Internal design and typesetting by Jude Rowe, Agave Creative Group
Illustrations by Johanna Roberts and Cristian Enache
First Aid Quick Reference section designed by grafica
Author photograph by Jason Malouin
Printed and bound in Australia by McPhersons Printing Group
The papers used by HarperCollins in the manufacture of this book are a natural,
recyclable product made from wood grown in sustainable plantation forests. The fibre
source and manufacturing processes meet recognised international environmental
standards, and carry certification.

CONTENTS

FOREWORD

Every now and then I come across a 'must have' book for families. *A Life. A Finger. A Pea Up a Nose.* is certainly one of these. Drawing on her work as a paediatric emergency nurse, and her experience as a mum, Sarah Hunstead has written a fabulous first-aid and 'what to do' book that should be in every home.

The choices we make in those seconds after an accident or serious incident can save lives. But often as parents we simply have no idea what to do. *A Life. A Finger. A Pea Up a Nose.* explores the everyday things that can happen to our children in our homes. To know that help — both well informed and practical — is close by should be a seriously huge relief to everyone.

I wish this book could have been in my home when my adventurous lads were little — it will certainly be in my grandchildren's homes.

Well done, Sarah.

Maggie Dent
Author, educator, and parenting and resilience specialist

Our children are the world's tomorrow.
Our future. Our hopes. Our dreams. Our greatest investment.
Our legacy. Our contribution to humanity.

As the minders and role models of little people, we must have the skills to keep them physically and emotionally safe.

Confidence in parenting comes from skill and knowledge. Having basic skills in first aid and CPR ensures we can bravely and confidently follow our children as they explore the world.

This book will give you practical skills. Empowering skills. Life-saving skills. Skills that will enable you to confidently watch and encourage your children as they explore the world and take the risks that are essential for them to become brave and resilient.

This book is a gift and its message is clear: be brave enough to develop the skills that will allow you to be your child's greatest protector and to umbrella them as they learn to weather life's storms.

Today we buy prams, car seats, food, education and opportunity for our children. Why not also invest in knowledge and skills that could save a life? We know 'it takes a village to raise a child'. But it also takes a conscious decision on the part of that village to establish a skill set that will protect and respond to a child's acute healthcare needs.

I challenge you to develop the confidence to protect all of our children.

Kylie Stark
Paediatric Emergency Department Nurse Manager,
co-founder of CanTeen, and recipient of the Michelle Beets
Memorial Award for the advancement of children's health within NSW

INTRODUCTION

Kids are amazing. They are resilient, fascinating little humans who occasionally end up needing medical help when things go wrong — some more often than others! As a paediatric emergency nurse with 15 years under my belt, I've often thought that I've seen it all — the emergency department can be a pretty eye-opening place. But then another child will come in with yet another injury that will inspire wonder. It seems the I-probably-shouldn't-do-this-because-the-outcome-could-be-very-bad switch is missing in a lot of kids.

Before starting CPR Kids, our baby and child first-aid education program, my career saw me working with some amazing clinicians in some equally amazing hospitals. I also got to witness countless times when parents had applied first aid to their children's injuries — usually with makeshift equipment, such as an eye patch made from a sanitary pad: great initiative! These parents knew the difference good first aid would make to the outcome of their child's health.

Another thing that can make a big difference to the outcomes of sick children is when parents and carers recognise concerning signs and symptoms and get the right kind of medical help quickly. We don't always have our wise mum or grandma there with us when the kids are sick. Knowing what to look for is *important*; seeking the right medical help at the right time is *essential*.

I consider myself *so very lucky* to have the skills and knowledge to help my kids — even if it takes a fair amount of coercion! It means that when they do hurt themselves or become sick, I can treat their injuries effectively and know when they need further medical help. I realise working in paediatric emergency care might give me the edge here, but in sharing my knowledge and experience via this book, I'm confident that you will also know what to do.

As a nurse, I've collected many stories over the years, but there are a few that remain etched in my mind. One of my clearest first-aid memories is of a three-year-old called James* who was active and curious. James was playing in the backyard, while his father was in the kitchen, watching him through the window. It was winter and it had been raining heavily. James's dad turned away for only a minute and when he turned back he saw his son face-down in a water feature in their garden — a shallow bowl that was still wide enough for James to fall into.

James's dad was trained in CPR (cardiopulmonary resuscitation). He knew what he needed to do. He ran to his little boy and pulled him out of the water. James was already blue after less than 60 seconds. His dad started CPR immediately, and after hearing his shouts for help, neighbours called an ambulance. James was rushed to hospital, CPR continuing all the way. His little heart had effectively stopped beating for over 60 minutes, but the CPR, and of course the other medical treatment he received later, saved his life.

After being resuscitated, James had a long recovery in hospital. Today he is a healthy, active, bright boy with parents who are thankful every day for their son's life. James would have had a very different outcome had his dad not known CPR. His brain would have lacked vital blood and oxygen, which would have resulted in severe brain damage or even death.

It is vital that all families learn the basics of first aid and CPR. You never know, the child whose life you end up saving may be your own.

Sarah Hunstead

P.S. Thoughout *A Life. A Finger. A Pea Up a Nose*. I refer to 'your' child as 'she' and 'her'. It's only because I have two daughters. I hope you'll understand ... Boys, you are not getting away with anything!

*Not his real name.

Please visit our YouTube channel **www.youtube.com/ cprkidsTV** and the CPR Kids Facebook page **@CPRKids** to watch hands-on demonstrations of the first-aid information provided in this book.

HOW TO USE THIS BOOK

First aid and sick kids are a part of every family's journey. My aims in writing this book are to help make that journey a safe and happy one, and to give you the confidence to make decisions about your child's health.

In *A Life. A Finger. A Pea Up a Nose.* you will read plenty of stories and anecdotes. Some will make your hair stand on end, some will make you laugh and some will make you cry. But *all* of them will make you think about the health and safety of your kids.

The first-aid and illness information contained in these pages is sourced from current, evidence-based practice recommended by governing bodies. The **Resources** section at the back of the book provides articles, phone numbers and websites that will give you further detail and help you stay up to date. Any references within the text are given in full in the **References** section at back of book.

This book is designed to *complement* a first-aid course, because the reality of acquiring first-aid skills is that hands-on learning is crucial. First-aid class resources are listed in the **Resources** section. And remember, if your child has a chronic illness or special needs, you need to make sure you have an action plan from your paediatrician for when they are sick or injured. Each child is unique, so make sure you know about any specific treatment your child needs.

In this book, you will find lots of practical hints and tips on how to apply first aid to kids. It might be a relatively easy thing to put a sling or bandage on an adult, but doing that to a screaming two-year-old is an entirely different challenge. If you're having visions of trying to stuff an octopus into a string bag, I understand. But don't worry; follow the steps provided here and you and your child will calmly and confidently navigate all manner of mishaps.

Caring for the health of your child involves three main steps: prevention, recognition and response. It's all well and good to know what to do if your child is hurt, but what about prevention? There are lots of common-sense things you can do to help prevent illness and injury. That said, it's also important to remember that you cannot wrap your children in cotton wool. They are amazingly robust and need to get out into the world, climb trees and eat mud. Risk-taking is a childhood rite of passage — it is part of building a confident, resilient adult. Minor injuries are inevitable; you just need to know how to patch them up.

It's also essential that parents and carers recognise the signs and symptoms of illness and know where to seek appropriate help. This is not about the diagnosis; it's about recognising that something is different from normal and knowing what to do.

The **First Aid Quick Reference** colour section at the centre of this book is designed to give you a handy go-to summary of the most relevant information you need in an emergency. The RED FLAGS featured throughout this section list the particular signs and symptoms that indicate your child needs urgent medical help.

All the advice in *A Life. A Finger. A Pea Up a Nose.* follows a logical approach that will allow you to remain calm and remember the underlying principles of first aid: act quickly, preserve life and prevent further harm. One of the key messages I want to convey in this book is the importance of staying calm. Seeing an injured child, especially if it's your own, can unleash a torrent of emotion that can make you feel as though you are falling apart inside. But if your child sees you panic, she will panic even more. Stay calm, reassure your child that everything will be all right, and keep it together. Fall apart later over a glass of wine when the dust has settled.

I strongly suggest you do regular face-to-face CPR and first-aid training in addition to reading this book. The reason is very straightforward. In the world of healthcare, we are constantly finding better ways to do things. What was used as a treatment for an illness or injury in the past might be completely different from what's recommended now, because evidence has shown that there is a better way, or that the old way may in fact be harmful. If you want to know the best way to help your child, make sure you keep your knowledge current, especially if your child has special needs.

Always remember: do what you can with what you have around you. Improvise, think outside the square, and do no further harm.

PART 1

BABIES, TODDLERS & CHILDREN

BABIES 0 TO 12 MONTHS: WHAT THEY DO AND WHY

When I brought our first pink, screaming bundle of joy home from the hospital, my partner and I had no idea what to do. No idea at all. We kept waiting for someone to tell us how to make her stop crying and how to interpret all her needs and wants in a timely fashion. This didn't happen, but gradually we all got used to each other and, almost nine years later, our daughter is a healthy, happy kid. So we must have done something right. We also went back and had another one, but an instruction book definitely would have been welcomed with both of them!

Luckily for unsuspecting parents, babies don't tend to fall out of trees or run in front of cars. Since they are relatively immobile, it is unlikely you are going to need to apply first aid for a broken bone or bleeding lip. Babies, however, do come with their own set of potential problems. There is a massive amount of growth and development in the first year, from learning to roll and sit up, to crawling and pulling themselves up onto things. Some will even learn to walk before their first birthday.

The first time your baby suffers an injury or illness can be very upsetting. It's also often the first time parents realise their baby is changing developmentally. Think about the first time your baby rolled — was it (almost) off the bed or the change table? It is easy to put a newborn to sleep in the middle of your bed, and indeed many parents do sleep with their babies. Provided your baby is in a safe sleeping situation it is highly unlikely she will roll out. Baby walkers are another cause of falls. These have been banned in some countries due to the number of preventable injuries that occur during their use.

The leading cause of hospital admissions for babies under the age of one is respiratory infection ('Health of Children in Australia: A Snapshot, 2004–05'). This is followed by accidental falls, usually while being carried, or by falling from a bed ('Serious Childhood Community Injury in New South Wales 2009-10'). About 75 per cent of infant drowning cases occur in the bath ('A Picture of Australia's Children 2012').

One of the major fears parents have with a new baby is Sudden Infant Death Syndrome (SIDS), or 'cot death'. The sudden death of a baby, when there is no apparent cause, is now called Sudden Unexpected Death in Infancy (SUDI), which includes SIDS and fatal sleep incidents. A baby can die of SUDI at any time of the day or night, but most die quietly in their sleep. The number of deaths due to SIDS has been reduced by 80 per cent in Australia since 1989 when the SIDS and Kids safe sleeping campaign was introduced.

Today, SIDS and Kids is known as Red Nose. According to their recommendations, the best safe sleeping practices are as follows:

+ Provide a safe sleep environment night and day.
+ Sleep your baby on her back from birth, not on her tummy or side.
+ Sleep your baby with her head and face uncovered.
+ Keep your baby in a smoke-free environment before and after birth.
+ Sleep your baby in her own safe sleeping place in the same room as an adult caregiver for the first 6 to 12 months.
+ Breastfeed your baby.

Another source of mixed emotions (usually joy and anxiety) is introducing solids. Many parents are concerned about allergic reactions. You don't need to camp outside the emergency department at the first offer of peanut butter, you just need to know what to do if there is a reaction.

Choking is also up there on the list of mishaps that can affect babies; they stick everything in their mouths. Remember, gagging is normal; choking is not. See **Choking**, pages 121–130, for more information.

When it comes to illness, your baby can't tell you when she doesn't feel well. Often the first thing a parent notices when their baby is unwell is that she doesn't feed as well as normal, she is unsettled or she is sleeping more than usual. You know what 'normal' is for your child. If something is different from normal, this could be a red flag (see **The Generally Unwell Child**, pages 182–185, for more information).

For parents of babies, CPR is an *essential* skill. When unhealthy adults experience a cardiac arrest, the heart either stops or doesn't beat properly, and then after a while breathing stops. The reverse is often true in babies and children. They usually have healthy hearts, so in cases of life-threatening injury or illness, it is usually the breathing that stops first, then the heart.

Reading about CPR is one thing, but nothing replaces a hands-on course. There are many baby- and child-specific first-aid courses offered in Australia, so look for one in your area.

SUMMARY

+ The leading cause of hospital admissions in babies is respiratory infection, followed by accidental falls.
+ Follow the Red Nose safe sleeping guidelines.

HOW THE MIGHTY TODDLER FALLS

Toddlers (one- to three-year-olds) are amazing. With their large heads, they make it their mission in life to whack their noggins into all manner of objects, from the edge of the dining-room table to the one pole within a 300-metre radius. Unbelievable? Wait until you have one.

Toddlers turn their parents' hair prematurely grey, usually by taking spectacular tumbles, only to miraculously surface again with the briefest spell of tears before getting straight back into it.

Not surprisingly, the leading cause of hospitalisation in toddlers is falls ('Serious Childhood Community Injury in New South Wales 2009–10'). Rates of drowning, burns, and poisoning are also high in this age group, with about 60 per cent of drownings occurring in swimming pools ('A Picture of Australia's Children 2012').

Toddlers are risk-takers, and learn by seeing, smelling, touching and tasting their world. No matter how much you tell yours not to do something, you can pretty much guarantee she is going to do it. My sister-in-law didn't know whether to laugh or cry when she found her 15-month-old son dipping his sippy cup into the toilet water and drinking it. Relax, he's fine.

The concept of consequence is not part of a toddler's thought processes. Toddlers don't see the danger in climbing onto a table — they only think about how exciting it would be to see the world from up there and how much more fun it would be to jump off. They live in the moment … though now that I think about it, I know a few adults who live that way too! While some kids will learn after they've tried the risky behaviour once or twice, others just keep going back for more, regardless of the outcome.

The extreme variability in a toddler's emotions, usually from one minute to the next, is also to be admired (and preferably from a distance if that child that does not belong to you). It's remarkable how a happy, beaming toddler can transform into a screaming, tantrum-throwing banshee in a matter of seconds. Frustration is one of the key toddler emotions. A toddler desperately wants independence but gets frustrated when things don't happen as quickly as she would like.

I was very lucky with my first daughter, because tantrums didn't seem to be her thing. She appeared to learn very quickly that when I told her not to do something because it would hurt, it was probably best not to do it. Not so with daughter number two. I am sure she has a little personal radar that senses my anxiety when she goes to jump off something twice her height or fly down a hill on her scooter. The greater my concern, the greater her adrenaline rush. Then she goes back for more. If I could permanently secure her helmet to her head I would probably relax a bit more, but as it is I'll have to work on disguising my anguish!

Head injuries are very common in this age group, particularly once toddlers learn how to walk. Luckily enough, the most common scenario is that they end up sporting an 'egg' on the forehead, have a little cry, and just get on with what they were doing. A toddler's resilience outshines most adults' when it comes to injuries.

Toddlers get into everything. Nothing is off limits (to them). Parents need to keep their eyes on their toddlers, lest they climb up on the bookshelf or empty out the contents of somebody's purse. This constant vigilance can be truly exhausting. Parents of multiples: I salute you!

Because of the curiosity that toddlers possess, poisonings are also common. To a toddler, the bright colours of medicines and cleaning products must mean they are delicious, so down the hatch they go. Prevention is always better than cure, so keep everything out of reach. And put Great Aunt Mabel's handbag out of the way when she comes to visit. Neither of you wants your toddler examining the contents of her bag and thinking those blood-pressure pills or that frosty pink lipstick would be tasty.

Choking is also very common. Toddlers still think it's a good idea to put objects in their mouths and other orifices. I have seen Lego pieces, peas (see **Foreign Bodies**, pages 149–152), coins and many other small objects squeezed, pushed and poked into various places. Children running with objects in their mouths are an accident waiting to happen, whether it's a mouth injury or choking on the object. I will never forget the little girl who was running with a chopstick in her mouth before she stumbled and managed to spear her right tonsil with it. It was straight to the operating theatre for that one.

Drowning is another of the main causes of death in this age group. The importance of water safety cannot be overemphasised, and not just around swimming pools. In my career, I have seen more children who have drowned or nearly drowned in the bath, than in swimming pools. And in almost all of the drownings I have seen, there has been an adult relatively close by, and every single drowning has been silent. Read more in **Drowning** (see pages 136–143).

As adults, it is our job to ensure our toddler's world is as safe for her as possible. To quote my wise father: 'Children need enough rope to explore, but not enough to hang themselves with.'

SUMMARY

+ Toddlers learn by exploring.
+ Falls are the most common cause of injury.
+ Home safety is essential.
+ Prevention is better than cure, so keep dangerous objects out of reach or locked away.
+ Always practise good water safety.

LOOK MUM, NO HANDS!
KIDS AND WHAT THEY DO
TO THEMSELVES

Once they leave toddlerhood, children start to understand the meaning of consequence a little better. They soon learn that if you run into traffic, there is a high likelihood you will be hit by a car. Although this understanding develops further over the years, we all know that growing up doesn't necessarily equate with less risky behaviour, so adults always need to be on the alert.

Evidence suggests that children have poorer peripheral vision than adults and this could account for the many pedestrian accidents that affect children. They are also easily distracted. If they are playing footy and the ball bounces onto the road, they concentrate on retrieving the ball, not necessarily on the car that is coming their way.

Falls from playground equipment such as monkey bars and trampolines are almost a childhood rite of passage. And broken bones, scrapes and cuts are just going to happen. Usually when things go pear-shaped, all that is needed is a Band-Aid, some antiseptic and a big hug from Mum or Dad. However, being prepared with first-aid skills that are appropriate for kids is imperative — just in case.

Interestingly, in this age group, boys are more likely to be injured than girls. Boys do exhibit greater risk-taking than girls, but there are always exceptions to the rule ('Serious Childhood Community Injury in New South Wales 2009–10').

The most common causes of injuries in children aged 5 to 14 in Australia are transport accidents, falls and drowning. Even for kids who can swim, drowning is a risk. Many injuries are related to sports and playground equipment, with collisions being one of the main causes of injury in boys (www.carrsq.qut.edu.au).

As kids get older, encouraging them to use safety equipment can be challenging. If the cool kid next door doesn't wear a helmet when skateboarding, your impressionable 10-year-old may be reluctant to protect her head too. I can remember being teased when I was eight for wearing a stack hat. Those GenXers out there will remember the old stack hats. Big, bold and not very cool, unless of course you covered them in stickers that matched the colours of your Spokey Dokes. But I wore one anyway. And it saved my life. Here's how …

One morning, Mum sent me up to the corner shop on my bike to buy bread and milk. On the way back I had to cross a busy road, so I hopped off my bike and stepped out into traffic. I didn't see the car coming. Travelling at 60 kilometres per hour, it ploughed into me, smashed my roadster to smithereens and catapulted me into the air. I landed on my head, on top of the bonnet (and for any of you who have ever owned a Datsun, you would know the bonnet is pretty hard). My trusty stack hat cracked in half, but it saved my brain. I woke up in the middle of the road having lost control of my bladder and broken only my leg and collarbone. I was a very lucky girl. One of the witnesses went to get Mum, who quickly scooped me up, along with the bread and milk, and took me to our GP. He put a cast on my leg but didn't worry too much about my collarbone.

Looking back, this incident horrifies me. If that had happened to a child brought into an emergency department, they would be rushed into the resuscitation room and examined by the trauma team. Fortunately, though I survived to tell the tale, and if anyone teased me again about wearing my helmet, I told them this story. In doing so, I hope I convinced others to protect their heads.

On your child's early life journey, minor injuries are inevitable. Try to prevent the major ones with protective headgear and other equipment, and know what to do if a major accident occurs. And remember, kids can learn CPR and first aid too.

SUMMARY

+ Leading causes of injury in kids aged 5 to14 are transport accidents, falls and drowning.
+ Many injuries are sport- or playground-related.
+ Minor injuries are an inevitable part of childhood.
+ Protective equipment such as helmets saves lives.
+ Even kids who know how to swim can drown.

PART 2

CPR & CALLING FOR HELP

CPR

The ability to perform cardiopulmonary resuscitation is a skill every parent must have.

CPR involves compressing the chest (and therefore the heart and lungs) so blood can be pumped around the body, and blowing air through the nose and/or mouth to inflate the lungs. CPR is performed when a person's heart has either stopped or is beating ineffectively. The aim of CPR is to keep blood (and the oxygen within it) circulating to the brain and other vital organs.

Contrary to popular belief, CPR is not about bringing someone back to life. To be honest, you would be extremely lucky if the person woke up while you were performing CPR on them. CPR is about keeping the brain and other vital organs well supplied with blood and oxygen. If the brain lacks blood and oxygen for even a few minutes, brain damage or death is likely to occur.

Even though the principles of CPR are the same across all ages, the way it is performed varies according to age. When practising CPR, ages are generally broken down into three groups:

1. Baby (0–12 months)
2. Child (1–8 years)
3. Adult

There is a logical and easy way to remember the steps of basic life support: via the acronym **DRSABCD**. Think how your doctors (DRS) might remember the basics of their job (ABCD). These letters stand for:

Danger
Response
Send for help
Airway
Breathing
Compressions
Defibrillator

DRSAB is about ascertaining whether or not somebody needs CPR, and CD is the performing of the CPR and defibrillation.

Let's look at each of the different components of DRSABCD in turn.

D – DANGER

You must check for danger before helping your child. This is easier said than done, because your parental instinct will kick in and your primary focus will be on aiding your hurt child immediately. But look at it this way: if you're also hurt, you can't help your child. So, you need to make sure that both you and your child are safe from any potential or further danger.

A good example of this is the story of a grandfather who saw his toddler grandson fall into a pool. Grandpa dived in after him, but couldn't swim. Mum then had to rescue both her son and her father. Luckily they were both fine in the end, but it was a double whammy that the mother didn't need. Though he had good intentions, Grandpa should have called for help, bless him.

Another example of this is when a parent runs out into traffic to rescue their child who has been hit by a car. The parent is not thinking clearly, so fails to look for oncoming traffic and is hit by another vehicle. Imagine receiving a phone call from the emergency department informing you that your child and partner have both been in an accident!

Take a moment to make sure you are safe, for your child's sake as well as your own. Then you need to make sure that your child is safe. Remember, if your child is injured, it is important to keep her still if possible (don't force her). However, if she is in danger where she is, it is a priority to move her out of the way of any further harm.

Once you have made sure you and your child are safe, move on to the next step.

R — RESPONSE

You need to know if your baby or child is responsive (conscious) or unresponsive (unconscious). If she is responsive, she does not need CPR. She might still be very sick and need an ambulance, with lights and sirens all the way, but she doesn't need you to do compressions on her chest.

If a baby or child is unresponsive, she'll be floppy and heavy, and won't move or make normal noises when you try to rouse her. Unconsciousness is different from sleeping. Sleeping is a natural state that your baby or child can be woken out of (sometimes needing a lot of stimulation if she's in a deep sleep), whereas a baby or child who is unconscious doesn't wake up or make deliberate movements when stimulated.

Most first-aid guidelines will tell you that unless an injured person is in danger, you should leave them where they are while checking for a response. The reason for this is that you may exacerbate an injury if you move them. The exception to this is when you need to keep the airway open — more on that in 'A – Airway' (see pages 34–37).

To check for responsiveness in a child, squeeze her shoulders firmly and give her a good tickle. Talk to her loudly, for example: 'Sarah, wake up Sarah, can you hear me?' Hopefully you will get a cry, or she will push you away or talk to you. This is good! She may still need urgent medical attention but she does not need CPR.

As a parent, I can't imagine leaving a baby in a cot and squeezing her shoulders to see if she is responsive. Pick up your baby, unless of course she has been in a car accident or a fall and you need to keep her still. While holding her upright in your arms and supporting her head, give her ribs a good strong tickle. Really stimulate her, but do not shake her. Hopefully you will get a cry.

Crying is good. A crying child does not need CPR.

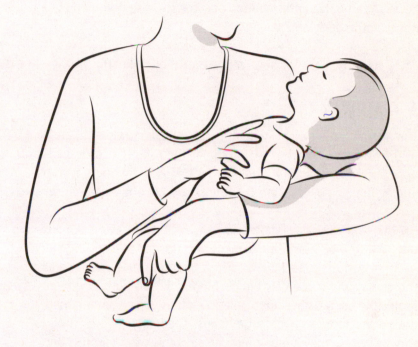

Checking for a response in a baby

A mum in one of my classes told us what happened when her very young baby lapsed into unconsciousness. She said at first she thought he was just in a deep sleep, but realised when she picked him up and tried to stimulate him that he was extremely floppy and did not give the little jerks that he normally did when he was picked up while asleep.

If your child or baby does not respond — that is, if she is unconscious — you need to move on to the next step.

S — SEND FOR HELP

If your baby is unresponsive, you need to get help any way you can, as quickly as possible (see **Calling 000**, pages 52–60). You might call 000 yourself, get someone who is with you to call an ambulance, bang on neighbours' doors or flag down a passing car. Whatever you decide, just do it.

If you call 000, stay calm and talk clearly. Don't forget to unlock doors, open gates and clear any obstacles so the paramedics can get to you quickly and safely.

Once you have sent for help, move on to the next step.

A — AIRWAY

The airway is the passageway through which air passes in and out of the lungs. The trachea (windpipe) is the tube that connects your nose and mouth to your lungs, and it needs to be open. If your airway is blocked, you stop breathing and life ends. It's that simple.

For babies, the airway is soft and narrow. If your baby is unconscious due to illness or injury, her muscles and normal reflexes are inactive, so if her head falls backwards or tips too far forward, this can kink the airway and cause very big problems. By comparison, the airway in healthy babies stays open, even when asleep. As mentioned, babies and toddlers have large heads. Their large heads can flop forward when they are unconscious and this can compress and block off the airway. Babies and toddlers also have large tongues. You can't actually swallow your tongue, but when you are *unconscious* due to illness or injury (*not* sleeping) the tongue flops back over the entrance to the airway, blocking it off.

Your baby's head needs to be placed in a neutral position in order to keep the airway open. This involves a manoeuvre called a head tilt chin lift.

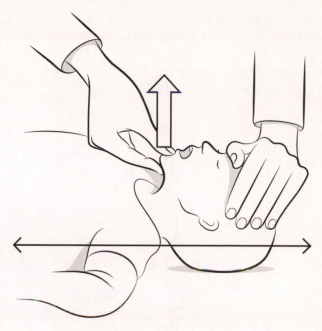

Neutral position in a baby

If she isn't there already, and providing it's safe to do so, put your baby or child on the floor. Move her head into a straight line with the rest of her body. A good way to understand this position is to do it yourself. Sit upright with the nice straight yoga spine we should all have. Look directly forward. This alignment of the head with the body is the neutral position you need to put your baby in. Once your baby's head is in the neutral position, using your thumb and index finger, lift her chin up towards the ceiling or sky.

As you do this be careful not to press on the soft parts around her throat, as this can also block the airway. The reason you need to lift her chin up is because this pulls her tongue forward, unblocking the entrance to her airway.

A child's head needs to be positioned differently from a baby's: it needs to be tilted back to open the airway. Using the head tilt chin lift, gently pull your child's head back. It's a bit like the position you take when you sniff something. A good way to describe this is to imagine you are sitting upright with the straight yoga spine again.

Pretend you have a bunch of flowers in your hands in front of you and lean forward to sniff them. Using your finger and hand, grasp your child's chin and lift it towards the ceiling. As for a baby, you are positioning the head and neck in a way that pulls the tongue forward to unblock the entrance to the airway.

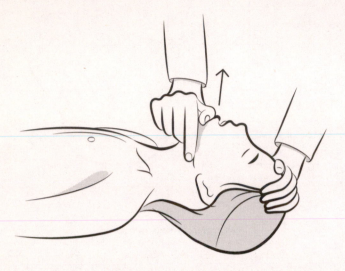

Head tilt chin lift in a child

You need to remember that with an unconscious baby, child or adult, airway opening takes priority over an injury. Even if you suspect that your child has hurt her neck or spine, you still need to tilt her head back to keep her airway open. Yes, you might exacerbate her injury (although this is unlikely), but if her airway is not open, she cannot breathe. If a baby has an object in her mouth that you can see when you open the airway, roll her onto her side, and if you can easily get it out, do so. If the object is right at the back, sweeping with your fingers may push the object further down — so don't sweep! If she has vomit in her mouth, roll her onto her side, let it drain out and then roll her back.

I once attended an accident in which a motorbike rider was hit by a truck. I followed DRSABCD, and when it came to assessing the rider's airway, I saw he was not doing well. His airway was blocked and he needed me to hold it open so he could breathe. In an unconscious person, if you let go of the head tilt chin lift, their head will usually flop back and the airway will become blocked again, so you need to keep holding it open. While I was doing this, I had a bystander yelling at me because he could see bones sticking out of the injured man's arm and a huge amount of blood. What the bystander didn't understand was why I was holding this man's head. Yes, he was bleeding heavily, but if I'd let go of his head, he would have stopped breathing. It didn't take long for other people to turn up, and someone else applied first aid to his arm while I kept holding his airway open until the ambulance arrived.

Once you have the airway open, keep holding and move on to the next step.

B – BREATHING

While you keep holding the airway open, you need to check for breathing. Even though the unconscious person still takes the occasional shallow gasp, this doesn't count as breathing. You need to look, listen and feel for normal or abnormal breathing.

+ Look for rise and fall of the chest or tummy.
+ Listen for sounds of breathing.
+ Feel for air coming out of the mouth or nose.

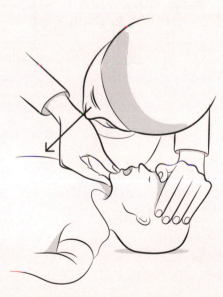

Look, listen and feel for breathing

You know what *normal* breathing looks like — you see it every day in your child. When you watch young babies breathe, you'll notice that they don't breathe regularly and their tummies rise and falls rather than their chests, as in adults and older children. When babies and children are breathing normally, they are pink — sometimes pale if they are unwell. But when they are breathing *abnormally*, they can turn blue very quickly, sometimes within 30 seconds of the start of abnormal breathing. This is one of the signs that a baby or child needs CPR.

If the baby or child is breathing *abnormally*, you might only see the occasional shallow gasp, or nothing at all. The baby or child will also be blue, which usually starts on and around her lips then spreads over her face and body. Her arms and legs will become mottled — the look your skin gets on a very cold day: splotchy or marbled. If a baby or child has dark skin, you will see her lips, nails and the inside of her mouth turn blue.

You may get to this stage and find that your child is unconscious but breathing *normally*. Think of a football player who's been knocked out on the field but doesn't require the medics to rush out and apply CPR. Similarly, a child who is unconscious but breathing normally will not require CPR but will need to be rolled into the recovery position (see **Recovery Position**, pages 48–51).

So, if your baby or child is unconscious, has abnormal breathing and is blue, you need to go on to the next step: commencing compressions.

UNCONSCIOUS + ABNORMAL BREATHING = COMPRESSIONS

Never do CPR on a conscious person. Not only will they be very cranky with you because it hurts, but if they are conscious they also don't need it.

C – COMPRESSIONS

The aim of doing compressions is to compress the rib cage over the heart and lungs to squeeze the blood out and circulate it around the body. As you release the compression, you allow the rib cage to rise and the heart to fill with blood again. And repeat! You are the pump.

One of the most common things that goes wrong in CPR is when the person performing the compressions does not go deep enough. It is very important to ensure that you compress to one-third of the depth of the chest. This is approximately four centimetres on a baby, five centimetres on a child and a minimum of five centimetres on an adult.

When performing CPR, the correct position for your hands or fingers is on the lower half of the breastbone (otherwise known as the sternum).

If you are not strong enough to compress to one-third of the depth of a child's chest with one hand, use two.

To compress the chest, put your baby or child on the floor. You must have a hard surface under your child or you will not be able to compress her chest deeply enough. If your baby or child is on a soft couch, for example, you will bounce her rather than achieving a decent compression depth.

Place your fingers or hand on the lower half of the breastbone. A good way of finding this in a baby or child is to imagine a line running across the chest between her nipples. This is the middle of the sternum. Put your hand just below this line for the compressions. For obvious reasons this does not work on adults, particularly women!

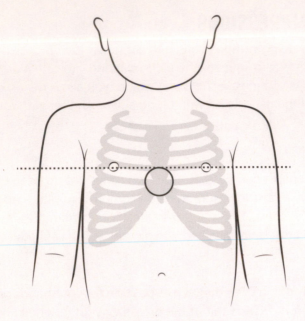

Position to do compressions

When you are ready to start compressions, kneel close to the baby or child, put your fingers or hand/s in position and lock your elbows. Don't make your arms do all the work; use your body. You will find that you can continue compressions for much longer this way. If you lean back and make your arms do all the work, you will tire very quickly and your compressions will not be effective.

Compressions should be smooth and rhythmic, but they are not easy, especially on an adult. It is a big physical workout and very tiring.

It is most important to make sure you let the chest come all the way up between compressions to allow the heart to fill up with blood again. Imagine the heart is a sponge, the large kind that you might use to wash a car. If you just gave a little squeeze, how much water would come out? Not much. Again, if you squeezed it really, really fast over and over again, not much water would come out. Now, if you gave it a good hard squeeze, then fully released it in more water, not only would you squeeze a big amount of water out of the sponge, but the sponge would also fill up with a big amount of water when let go. The same goes for the heart.

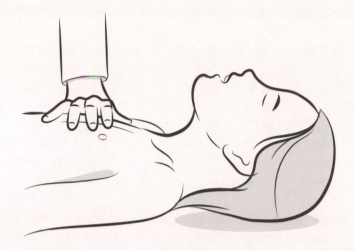

Compression depth is one-third of the depth of the chest

You need to aim for 100 to 120 compressions per minute (two compressions per second). Coincidentally, this is the rhythm of the Bee Gees song 'Stayin' Alive'. 'Baa Baa Black Sheep' also works and, for our friends in the UK, so does 'Nelly the Elephant'. This compression rate is the same for babies, children and adults.

+ Depth: one-third the depth of the chest
+ Speed: 100 to120 compressions per minute ('Stayin' Alive')
+ Position: Lower half of the breastbone
+ Ratio: 30 compressions to two breaths

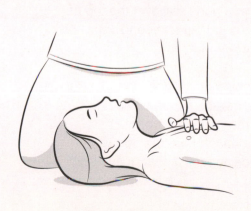

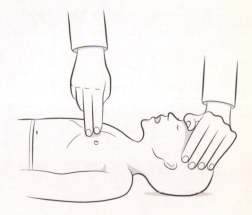

One or two hands for a child   *Two fingers for a baby*

You have probably heard about compression-only resuscitation (no giving of breaths, just compressions). However, in CPR there is a breaths component, known as mouth-to-mouth resuscitation. If an adult requiring CPR is close to help (say, in a metropolitan area), there is medical evidence to show that compression-only resuscitation will still be of benefit, as there is enough oxygen already present in the blood to supply the brain for the relatively short time it will take for help to arrive. Mouth-to-mouth is not an easy thing to do and the evidence says that we should not waste time attempting it in such cases. Rather, for an adult, it is best to keep the blood circulating with compression-only resuscitation.

That said, in Australia we are still teaching mouth-to-mouth for a few reasons. First, much of our population is rural so it can be some time before professional medical help arrives. Also, mouth-to-mouth is very important in resuscitating someone who has drowned. When it comes to babies and children, the evidence clearly states that giving mouth-to-mouth is very important. My view is that if you can give mouth-to-mouth, do so. If for some reason you can't, for example if you are heavily pregnant, you have breathing difficulties, or the person is injured and covered in blood, protect yourself and do compressions only.

Rather than doing mouth-to-mouth resuscitation on babies, it is much easier to do mouth-to–mouth-and-nose resuscitation. This involves putting your mouth over the baby's mouth and nose, making sure you have a good seal. You can use this method on a baby until she is too big for you to get a good seal over the top of her mouth and nose. For a child who is too big for you to apply this method, you will need to do mouth-to-mouth.

When you do mouth-to-mouth breathing on anyone, don't forget to block off the nose. If you breathe into the mouth without blocking off the nose, the air will come straight out of the nose rather than going into the lungs. Another important thing to remember during this procedure is to keep the airway open using the head tilt chin lift. Remember, if the airway is blocked or kinked, the air cannot get into her lungs.

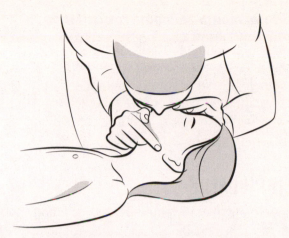

Mouth-to-mouth breathing on a child

Think about the size of a baby's or child's lungs in relation to yours. An adult's lungs are substantially bigger. As a general guide, a newborn needs only a puff of air. A baby needs the air volume of your distended cheeks — purse your lips and puff out your cheeks like a bullfrog; it looks a bit silly but that is about how much air is needed to inflate a baby's lungs. A child will take more, depending on her size.

Once you have opened up the airway and blocked off her nose (if you're not doing mouth-to–mouth-and-nose), put your mouth over hers and ensure you have a good seal. Breathe into her mouth. As you are doing this, watch her chest. If you see it rise, you have delivered enough air. Take your mouth off to let her breath come out, then repeat.

Give two breaths and then recommence your compressions. If you are turning beet-red and forcing air in, it is probably too much. You don't want to cause lung damage, so ease off on the force of your breath.

The ratio of compressions to breaths is 30:2. Remember, it is two attempts at giving breath — don't waste your time doing extra breaths if you think the first ones haven't worked. The most important part is the compressions.

How to perform mouth-to-mouth resuscitation

+ Open the airway using the head tilt chin lift.
+ Ensure you have a good seal over the mouth or mouth and nose.
+ Breathe into your child or baby.
+ Take your mouth off to let her breath come out.
+ Breathe into her again.
+ Ratio is 30 compressions to two breaths.

D — DEFIBRILLATOR

AEDs are now found in many public places, including shopping centres, schools, office buildings, train stations and gyms. AEDs save lives, and if one is available it should always be usedas part of DRSABCD. You do not need to be trained to use a defibrillator, just follow the pictures and prompts on the box and listen to what the machine tells you to do. A defibrillator can be used on

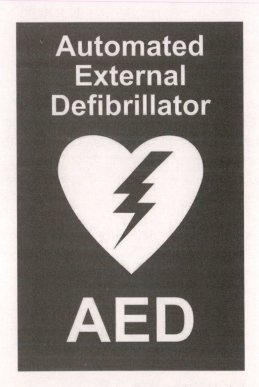

You know on television when they yell 'Stand clear!' and give the patient a shock to put their heart in the right rhythm? Those things are called Automated External Defibrillators (AEDs)

everyone — babies, children and adults. Even if you only have adult pads available, you can still put them on a child. Just make sure the pads are not touching each other. If you are by yourself, don't stop doing compressions to retrieve a defibrillator, but please do get one if there is more than one person present. One of you can continue the compressions and one can attach the AED.

Make sure you attach the sticky pads to bare skin, turn on the machine and just listen. The AED will only give a shock if the person actually needs it — it is automated!

WHEN DO YOU STOP CPR?

+ When your baby or child starts responding to you (becomes conscious).
+ When medical help arrives and takes over (most likely scenario).
+ When you are too physically exhausted or it is too dangerous to keep going.
+ When an AED tells you to stop.

If you're in a metropolitan area, it is likely that the paramedics will arrive and take over before you become too exhausted.

It is really important that you learn hands-on CPR. Even though you will gain an understanding from reading this book, nothing replaces the hands-on practice. Pick a course in which you get lots of practical time on baby and child mannequins so you can get a feeling for what it would be like to perform CPR on a real baby or child. This will help commit the information to your memory, and 'muscle memory', so that in an emergency you will be able to recall what to do and do it well.

BASIC LIFE SUPPORT

D   **Dangers – are there any?**

R   **Response – is your child unresponsive?**

S   **Send for Help**

A   **Airway – is it open?**

B   **Breathing – is it abnormal?**

C   **CPR**
30 compressions to 2 breaths
If unwilling/unable to perform rescue breaths continue chest compressions

D   **Defibrillator – attach AED**
as soon as available and follow its prompts

Continue CPR until child responds or normal breathing returns

Basic life support — DRSABCD

'The most terrifying seven minutes of my life'

We had just arrived in Melbourne to visit my in-laws. Our boys were chasing each other around the dining table, laughing. As they laughed and played, my husband took Ravi, our 22-month-old, in his lap and started feeding him lunch. Ravi suddenly started staring off into space and became completely unresponsive. I started shouting his name. Still no response. I grabbed him from my husband, and by now Ravi was floppy like a rag doll. I checked he wasn't choking on anything and screamed at my husband to ring 000. He and my mother-in-law stood motionless with shock. I put Ravi in the recovery position, checked his vital signs and then spoke to the woman on 000. My mother-in-law was making the situation more stressful, so I sent her outside to wait for the ambulance. My husband was still in shock.

Ravi's breathing had slowed, was barely perceptible and he was clammy. He then stopped breathing, turned blue and I couldn't feel his pulse any more. I thought my baby had died. I was freaking out inside, but fortunately as a dentist I am trained in advanced life support and CPR, and we do refresher courses regularly.

This meant I just switched onto autopilot and started CPR on Ravi. I kept telling myself to keep it together. After some compressions and breaths, Ravi started breathing again, his colour began to return to normal, and then soon after the ambulance arrived. I had him back in the recovery position and could hear him faintly saying 'Mama'.

All of this happened over seven minutes — the most terrifying seven minutes of my life. It highlighted to me that most people don't know First aid or CPR. Literally, my husband and mother-in-law had no idea what to do. We spent our holiday in Melbourne at the hospital. After many tests we still don't have a definitive diagnosis, but thankfully we now have a healthy, happy two-year-old. Briefly, I didn't think we would.

On returning home, I organised for my husband and everyone who's in close contact with my kids to do a CPR Kids and first-aid course. It was invaluable, and we are all now equipped with the skills to help if an emergency arises again. Obviously, we're hoping to never have to use those skills, but I'm so grateful we have them.

Nitu

RECOVERY POSITION

The recovery position is the position in which you should place an unconscious or semiconscious child who is breathing normally. Placing your child on her side drains vomit or other fluid out of her mouth and keeps her airway open to help with breathing while you wait for medical help. There are many ways to do this, but it's important to be gentle if you are concerned your child may have a neck or back injury. Even if you suspect your child is injured, if she is unconscious but breathing normally you MUST put her on her side.

It doesn't matter which way you roll your child, the important points to remember are:

+ She should be on her side.
+ The position should be stable.
+ Avoid pressure on her chest.
+ Be aware of the need to roll her gently in case of spinal injury.
+ Be able to watch her.
+ The position should not injure her.

PLACING YOUR CHILD OR BABY IN THE RECOVERY POSITION

For a child over the age of one, or who is too heavy for you to hold safely, follow the steps illustrated:

1.

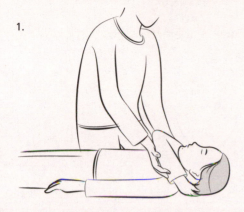

Place her hand under the side of her face.

2.

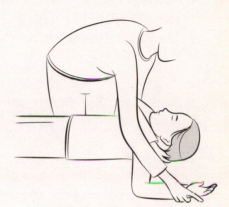

Move her other arm away.

3.

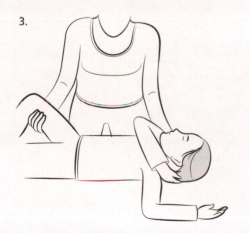

Lift your child's knee and place your other hand under her shoulder. Roll her gently away from you.

4.

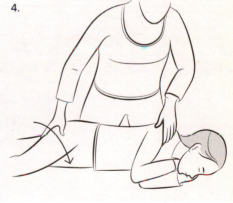

Lift her knee up to 90 degrees. Check that her hand is still under her face and ensure the airway is in the right position for her age (see pages 34–36).

How to place a child in the recovery position

For a small baby less than one year old and light enough to safely hold (be aware she will be heavy and floppy when unconscious), follow these steps:

+ Pick up your baby carefully.
+ Hold her jaw with your hand and place her body tummy-down along your arm.
+ Keep her head in line with her body — the neutral position (see **CPR**, pages 30–47).
+ Make sure she is facing downwards.

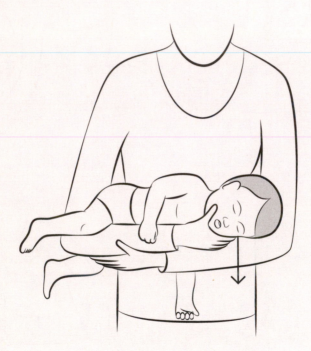

Holding a baby in the recovery position

Watch a demonstration of this, and other procedures covered in this book, on our YouTube videos at **www.youtube.com/cprkidsTV**.

'Ghostly white, cool to touch and like a rag doll in my arms'

When my daughter Taylor was six months old, she came down with a fever. It was clear she was pretty miserable, so I gave her some paracetamol as per the packet directions and stayed with her till she settled down, before going to bed myself. The next day I woke up at 6.30 a.m. and jumped out of bed thinking, 'My God, it's late!' I went into Taylor's room to check on her, only to find her ghostly white, cool to touch and like a rag doll in my arms. I was a paramedic at the time and recognised these symptoms. I knew something was very wrong. I raced into the kitchen where my mum was (she was staying with us at the time) and immediately gave Taylor to her. Once she was out of my arms I was able to calm down and think about how to handle the situation. She was having a febrile convulsion. I quickly put her in the recovery position, refraining from hugging her or following any other motherly instinct. I then called an ambulance.

After that first one, Taylor had a few more convulsions and I got better at dealing with them. As a mum, I found the situation incredibly frightening, but as a paramedic and someone who is trained in first aid, I was able to deal with the situation relatively calmly. I saw the red flags, but another mum or dad might not have, which is why it is so important that adults are trained in first aid.

Melanie
Paramedic

CALLING 000

When someone gets seriously sick or hurt, you call an ambulance. Sounds easy, doesn't it? But when something happens to your own child, calling for help may not be as straightforward. Panic can set in and your brain seems to temporarily exit your body. Too many times I have seen or heard about a situation where someone has forgotten the number to call, can't tell the operator where they live or has been too hysterical to actually tell the operator what is going on. Panic delays help, but if it's an emergency, you want that ambulance's lights and sirens on the way to you, pronto.

In Australia, the number to call for emergency services is 000.

Calling 000 will connect you to an operator who will ask if you need the 'police, fire or ambulance'. Even with no reception or zero credit left on your mobile phone, you can call 000. You need to be calm and clear when you speak to the operator. The more clearly you say where you are and what is wrong, the sooner help will be directed to you. Stay on the phone. Do not hang up until the operator tells you to. They can talk you through CPR and first-aid treatment.

The international standard emergency number is 112.

112 is the best number to call from a mobile phone when you're overseas and you don't know the area's emergency services number. Most countries use this as a secondary emergency number, so when

one of the kids has edged a bit too close to the fire dancing on your tropical holiday, calling 112 from a mobile phone should connect you to emergency services.

The average response time in urban areas of Australia for life-threatening emergencies is 10 minutes or less. Paramedics are highly skilled professionals but they rely on you to provide an accurate history of what has happened and any treatment you have already given, so being calm is essential. Most importantly, tell them if your child has any allergies.

In one of my first-aid classes we heard a mum speak about the time her newborn son stopped breathing. She said that she had put him down to sleep, but five minutes later had a funny feeling that something was not right, so she went in to check on him. She found him blue and barely breathing. She said she initially panicked, picked him up and started screaming. She then realised that she needed to get it together quick-smart and find help. With no idea where her phone was at that moment, the quickest way she could think of to get help was to run into the foyer of her apartment building, bang on doors and scream. Very quickly her neighbours came, one calling an ambulance and another commencing CPR. This mum did the right thing. Instead of wasting time looking for her phone, she got help the quickest way she knew how — and it worked. Sometimes the quickest way to get help is to have someone else call 000 for you.

One thing that you must always remember is this:

000 is for emergencies only!

If your child has a cold or has just vomited up her lunch, calling 000 is not appropriate. You are tying up essential services that other people with life-threatening illnesses or injuries need. Call your GP or local health advice line (see **Resources**, pages 233–239) and save 000 for emergencies only.

And if you're in an emergency situation, always call 000!

Make sure the paramedics have clear, direct access to where you are. Unlock doors and gate, or take your child and go outside if it's safe to do so. Alternatively, send someone else outside to wait for the paramedics to arrive.

Do not attempt to drive to the hospital. I recall a child who arrived at hospital having had a seizure. His mum panicked and put the child into the car and set off for the hospital, which was only five minutes' drive away. On the way, her child started having another seizure. Mum of course stopped suddenly, nearly causing a five-car pile-up. Another motorist called an ambulance.

So, even if you are only a few minutes away from the hospital, you need to consider what happens if your child stops breathing while in the car. How will you do CPR? You're better to wait 15 minutes for an ambulance at home doing effective CPR than spend five minutes in the car with no CPR.

If you're thinking of driving an injured child to hospital, it's unsafe to do so if:

+ You are unable to put your child in her child seat due to her illness or injury.
+ Your child's breathing is affected.
+ There is a possibility your child's illness or injury could become life-threatening.

For any of the above, call an ambulance. Even if you are not completely sure about whether to call an ambulance or not, do it. Trust your instincts.

The **Emergency+** app for smartphones is well worth downloading. It uses the GPS in your smartphone to pinpoint your location, so you can tell emergency services exactly where you are. This is particularly important if you are bushwalking, or even just visiting friends in an area you are unfamiliar with.

Kids need to learn how to call 000 too. When I was four years old, my mother collapsed and I needed to call for an ambulance. I knew to call 000 and tell them my address. When my girls were three- and four-year-olds both loved playing the 000 game. They can recite their address and know the importance of getting help quickly. Just be prepared to intervene if they decide to try it out for real. Yep, been there. The Triple Zero website (**www.kids.triplezero.gov.au**) has many games and resources to help kids to learn how and when to call 000.

SUMMARY

+ Call 000 for emergency services only.
+ Stay CALM and CLEARLY state where you are and what is wrong.
+ Get help the fastest way possible, any way you can.
+ Make sure the paramedics can access where you are, or send someone to wait for them.
+ Always call an ambulance in an emergency — do not drive to the hospital.
+ Teach your kids how to call emergency services.

What to expect when you call 000

As soon as babies start to crawl, the injuries begin. When they advance to eating solids, your lovingly prepared meals are thrown at the wall and instead babies want to eat playdough/paint/pages of books … or anything with a warning label. And as soon as they start playing with other kids, welcome to the world of snot and chest infections!

Over the last 16 years working as a paramedic, I have been involved in the treatment of children with all sorts of illnesses and injuries. Some serious, some not so much.

If your child is seriously hurt, you KNOW to call an ambulance. When your child is sick, however, it can be a little more confusing knowing when to call.

Raising a child can be overwhelming at the best of times. Sometimes my own little girl seems like another species. Nobody can quite prepare you for the challenges and worries you sometimes face when you're looking after a sick child, but nobody knows a child as well as her parents or her primary carer. So if you are concerned, call an ambulance.

When you call 000 (that's right, it is not 911) you will be transferred to an ambulance operator and they will ask for your details. We need to know where you are. As soon as an address is known and just a little information on your child's condition, an ambulance will be dispatched.

The call will then continue and the operator will go through a series of questions to gather as much information as possible. They will also offer advice on how to help your child until the arrival of the paramedics (the ambulance). The operator can talk you through what to do if your child is having a seizure, if they have fallen and been injured, or even talk you through CPR if needed. So, if at all possible, keep calm and stay on the line. An ambulance IS on its way to you!

When the ambulance arrives, the paramedics will come into your home to help you and your child. Be aware we may ask you to turn off the episode of Peppa Pig blaring from the TV, and possibly to lock the curious/noisy dog away in another room before he starts munching on our legs. We need to ask questions and gather as much information as possible. Gone are the days of an ambulance being merely a means of transport — paramedics are highly trained clinicians who can rapidly assess your child and initiate pain relief or life-saving treatment.

To a paramedic, the best sound in the world is a crying child. We are more concerned when a child is quiet, floppy or unresponsive. If your child is really unwell, we may initially be really busy looking after her. As soon as we can, we will talk to you and keep you informed of her condition and what we are doing.

If it is not a life-threatening situation, we will thoroughly assess your child and inform you of all our findings. Some conditions may require transport to hospital and others may be okay to treat and leave in your care. If the latter is the situation, do not feel silly. It is the very best outcome. And we don't pass judgement — we know how quickly a child can roll off/trip over/fall from/run into something. It's best to get them assessed by paramedics, and potentially a doctor, if you have any concerns.

If your child requires transport to hospital, you will most likely go with her in the ambulance. Grab her favourite toy (your phone also works well for distraction and entertainment). Your child may either love or be suspicious of their paramedic. She will not be a fan if the paramedic needs to perform any procedures like an injection or intravenous (IV) cannula, but these will only be performed where necessary. So, sit back, give your child a big hug and we will do our best to make them feel better.

Sally
Intensive care paramedic

'Follow your instincts'

When my daughter Abby was around nine months old, we were hosting a barbecue at our house. I asked my husband to watch over her while I had something to eat. She fell out of her pram and hit the base of her skull on the edge of the house. She started crying immediately and for a long time was completely inconsolable. Though crying is usually a good sign in injured babies, I decided to call an ambulance to be safe. Abby was soon treated at the Gold Coast Hospital and made a full recovery. Parents often worry about calling 000 for help, but when it comes to kids, it is better to be safe than sorry. When Abby was injured, I went with my gut feeling and called the ambulance. If you are worried about your child, you are usually right. If everything turns out to be fine then so be it — nothing has been lost and you run no risk of making things worse for your kid. As a parent, you should always follow your instincts.

Melanie
Paramedic

'I had to remain calm and strong for him'

One thing I learned from my son's accident is that you cannot rely on maternal instinct alone in an emergency. If I had, I would have swept my injured son straight off the road and into the comfort of my arms, potentially breaking his neck and back. I would have spent my time crying rather than reassuring. Fortunately, my first-aid training gave my shock and adrenaline a place to go that was practical rather than emotional.

About a year ago, I was paying the restaurant bill after a family dinner while my husband took our two sons to our car. Suddenly I heard the sound of my two-year-old, Arlo, screaming in a way that I had never heard before. I couldn't see him — I didn't need to. I knew it was bad so I yelled out 'Call an ambulance!' As I ran out of the restaurant I saw him on the road by the wheel of a four-wheel drive.

Fortunately, by the time I reached Arlo, he was already being supported by two men, in case of a spinal injury. I did not ask any questions, there was no time for that. I just dropped to my knees beside him. I must have landed hard, as later I noticed my knees were bleeding. I put my head over his and I said firmly, 'It's Mummy, you are going to be okay.' His injuries were severe and disturbing and nothing could have prepared me for the sight of his limbs, which had been crushed by the wheel. My initial thought was that he was going to lose his left arm and right hand. But that didn't matter to me. What mattered was that he lived — it was the first time in my life when I actually wanted him to cry.

Arlo's eyes kept darting from side to side, and I hoped it was from the intensity of his pain and shock and not from a head injury. I tried to speak calmly when I yelled out to the bystanders that he had lost his fingers and I needed something to stem the flow of blood.

When his cries became softer, I desperately wanted him to cry louder. The man beside me urged me to tell Arlo to stay with me, but instead I said to him, 'I love you', and suddenly I could feel my fear begin to overwhelm me. I remember my son's eyes stopped darting at that point. They stopped and looked vulnerably straight into mine; it was a look I will never forget. He was sensing my fear and it was frightening him, weakening him. In an instant I

pulled myself together and I said with absolute confidence, 'But you are going to be okay', and to my relief, his cries became loud again.

That look in Arlo's eyes was enough to tell me I had to remain calm and strong for him. It told me that despite his enormous pain and suffering, he was looking to me for comfort and reassurance. I wasn't there to take his tears away; I was there to keep them going.

We got to the hospital quickly, as a police car escorted our ambulance. When the doors to Emergency flew open, at least 10 medical staff were waiting for Arlo, and a social worker was waiting for me. She stood by in case I needed her. She also had to inform me that news crews had gathered outside the hospital but I said I wanted to keep Arlo's condition private. I wanted no distractions.

While Arlo's injuries were being assessed by the emergency doctors, I was given jobs that allowed me to be in his focus, such as holding the oxygen mask over his face. I distinctly remember looking down at my hands holding the mask and wondering why on Earth they weren't shaking when I was so terrified. Arlo gave me strength, because I knew that despite all his cries

Continued over page

of pain and amongst all the chaos of emergency surgeons and doctors, he was listening to me, so I just kept speaking. I told him about all the friendly people in funny uniforms who were looking after him and were going to make him better. I told him he was going to be doing some roly-polies when they had to turn him over. I told him stories from books we had read together, and when he had to go through the CAT scan machine I told him it was like a space ship.

As the doctors wheeled Arlo towards the operating theatre, he could only see the ceiling because he was in a neck brace, so my husband and I counted the fluorescent lights with him. For the first time, instead of a cry, came a little whisper from our son: 'Three, four, five.' And from that moment, I knew he was on the road to recovery. Three operations, two admissions to intensive care, ongoing hand and scar physiotherapy — he endured a lot for a little boy. But he has since made a full recovery, with his only permanent injury being to parts of his hand.

The only hero in Arlo's story is Arlo. But as his mother, I am grateful to the people who allowed me to stay by my son's side at a time when he needed me most; to the man on the road who I later found out was a policeman; and to my first-aid instructor whose words stayed with me throughout the most terrifying time of my life: 'Calm and reassure.'

We protect our kids with seat belts in cars, life jackets in boats and helmets on bikes. We acknowledge accidents can happen, so we should protect them with first aid too. If you never get to see the benefits of your course, please be grateful!

Eliza

PART 3

FIRST AID FOR COMMON INJURIES & SITUATIONS

ALLERGIC REACTION & ANAPHYLAXIS

Allergic reaction and anaphylaxis (life-threatening allergic reaction) are hot topics in healthcare circles. And rightly so. The prevalence of allergic reaction is significantly higher now than 30 years ago and it is estimated that one in three Australians has some form of allergy. Even more alarming is the news that one in 100 people will have anaphylaxis at some stage in their life. There is much groundbreaking research shedding light on the allergy epidemic, including the link between probiotics and gut health. It seems that it may be a combination of things, not one cause alone, so it's a case of constantly staying informed, particularly if you or someone you know suffers from allergies.

When a child is allergic to a particular food or substance — such as dust mites, pollen or insect stings — and is exposed to it, an allergic reaction occurs. When the substance (the technical term is allergen) enters the body via swallowing, inhalation or touch, the body's response is to produce antibodies. When the allergen comes into contact with the antibodies, the body's physiological response is to produce a number of substances, one of which is called histamine. The release of histamine into the body causes inflammation and swelling, the symptoms of allergic reaction. Reactions can range from mild to life-threatening.

Prevention

Kids can be allergic to a wide range of things, from insect stings to foods. The more common allergens include dairy, nuts and eggs. You don't need to camp outside the local emergency department when introducing these foods to your baby, just follow the guidelines provided below.

The Australian Society of Clinical Immunology and Allergy (ASCIA) now recommends the introduction of solids between four and six months of age, and it also recommends introducing foods that are known as highly allergenic before 12 months of age. Following these guidelines may help reduce the risk that your child will develop food allergies or eczema.

The summary below is taken from ASCIA's guidelines for introducing solids to infants. Stay up to date with their latest guidelines at **www.allergy.org.au**.

+ Introduce foods one at a time, around two days apart so that you can easily identify whether any foods cause a reaction. Allergic reactions usually occur quickly — from within minutes to two hours — while, in some, reactions may be more delayed.
+ All infants should be given foods in the first year of life that are common food allergens, including peanut butter, cooked egg, dairy and wheat products. This includes infants considered to be at high risk of developing food allergies.
+ ASCIA recommends introducing cooked egg and peanut butter in small amounts. Offer well-cooked egg and smooth peanut butter. You can do this by mixing a small amount of hardboiled egg or peanut butter (about ¼ baby spoon) into your infant's usual food such as vegetable puree, and gradually increasing the amount (up to several spoonfuls) if your infant is not having any allergic reactions.
+ Continue to include different foods so you can build a diet that contains a wide variety of foods. If a food causes a reaction, stop feeding your child that food and seek medical advice.

Introducing foods can be tricky if you have an older child who has allergies. You still need to introduce these foods to your baby, but you need to keep your other family member safe at the same time. Tips from ASCIA to tackle this issue include:

+ Introduce the food when the family member with the allergy is not at home.
+ Use separate cooking utensils to prepare and give the food to your infant, and wash them well afterwards.
+ Wash your and your infant's hands and face with soap after giving the food.
+ Offer the new food outside your home (for example at a relative's home) if you don't want to have the food in the house. Wash your and your infant's hands and face and ensure your and your infant's clothing is free of the food allergen before you return home.
+ Discuss with your dietitian how to introduce one child's allergen to another child in your family. As always, be aware of what to do if an allergic reaction occurs.

Recognition

It is important to be able to recognise the signs and symptoms of allergic reaction and anaphylaxis. Rubbing peanut butter or other foods into your child's skin won't help you figure out if they have an allergy. Your child's skin is very sensitive, so it may become red or irritated when it comes into contact with certain foods. Be mindful that this *may not be an allergic reaction*, just sensitivity. As always, it's best to check with your doctor.

Signs of **mild to moderate allergic reaction** include:

+ Swelling of the face or the area of an insect sting site
+ Hives or welts (rash) on the skin
+ Tingling mouth or lips
+ Unsettled/inconsolable behaviour (babies)
+ Abdominal pain and/or vomiting (these are signs of a mild to moderate allergic reaction to most allergens, but for insect allergy these are signs of anaphylaxis)

Signs of **anaphylaxis** (severe allergic reaction) include:

+ Difficult/noisy breathing
+ Swelling of the tongue
+ Swelling/tightness in the throat
+ Wheezing or a persistent cough
+ Difficulty talking and/or a hoarse voice
+ Persistent dizziness or collapse
+ Paleness and floppiness (babies and young children)

Response

For **mild to moderate allergic reactions**:

+ Stay calm.
+ Reassure your child.
+ Remove the food or substance, or flick out the sting.
+ For tick allergies, use a freezing spray to freeze-dry the tick and allow it to drop off (see also 'Ticks', pages 82–85).
+ Phone 000 for an ambulance.
+ Give medications (if prescribed by your child's doctor) or locate her adrenaline autoinjector (if she has one).

Continue to watch for any **one** of the signs of anaphylaxis as listed above. If **the reaction is severe or life-threatening**:

+ Lay your child flat. If breathing is difficult, allow her to sit on the floor with her legs out in front of her, but DO NOT let her stand up or walk around.
+ Use an adrenaline autoinjector if available.
+ Phone 000 for an ambulance.
+ Further adrenaline doses may be given if there is no response after five minutes.
+ If she becomes unconscious, follow basic life support — DRSABCD (see **CPR**, pages 30–47).

If your child has anaphylaxis, ensure your GP or paediatrician has provided you with an anaphylaxis action plan for her. Give this to your child's school or kindy and to other members of the family or people who regularly look after your child. Action plans, such as the one featured in the **First Aid Quick Reference** colour section, are available for download from the ASCIA website.

If you ever need to give a child her adrenaline autoinjector, make sure you read the pictorial instructions on the pen itself. It is better to delay giving the autoinjector by 15 seconds while you read the instructions and administer it in the correct way than to panic and give your child an ineffective dose, or worse, no dose at all. Always inject it into her thigh, preferably in the middle and on the side (you know, the meaty bit). You can even administer it through clothing — just make sure you hold it firmly in place as you do so.

If you are in any doubt about whether you need to administer the autoinjector, err on the side of caution. It is not going to do your child any harm if you administer it unnecessarily, but not doing so could mean death.

The adrenaline autoinjector available in Australia is EpiPen. There are both adult (EpiPen) and child (EpiPen Jr) versions. Anapen was discontinued in 2015, though a new model of Anapen has been released in Europe.

Remember, always trust your instincts — if you are concerned for any reason, seek medical help.

SUMMARY

+ Children can be allergic to a wide range of things.
+ Follow the ASCIA recommendations for introduction of solids (as summarised on pages 63–64).
+ Always follow your child's individual allergy or anaphylaxis action plan.
+ If you aren't sure about whether or not to administer your child's EpiPen, always err on the side of caution and give it!

Recognising symptoms of severe allergic reaction

My three-year-old daughter had never before shown signs of a severe allergic reaction. But one evening, as I was undressing her for a bath, I noticed a few red spots on her body. After the bath, they became more obvious and were appearing all over her. The bath water was pretty warm so I assumed the irritation would calm down as she cooled off but when my husband and I put her to bed, she seemed very restless and complained of being itchy. The red spots began to disappear and reappear on different parts of her body. She was evidently struggling to breathe and quickly became quite upset. Recognising these symptoms as signs of an allergic reaction, my husband and I decided it would best if he took her to the hospital for a check-up. She was seen quickly and given a dose of antihistamine. This immediately calmed her breathing and allowed the itchiness to settle down.

While we still don't know the cause of her irritation (she hasn't had another reaction since), we are glad we were able to recognise her symptoms and seek professional advice straight away.

Kristin

ASTHMA

Childhood asthma is very common in Australia. One in 10 Australians suffers from this potentially life-threatening condition. Fortunately, many children's symptoms can be controlled with good management and an asthma action plan. However, for some, asthma can be difficult to manage and can continue into adulthood.

Asthma is a long-term condition. When there is an asthma flare-up, the airways in the lungs become narrow due to swelling, muscle spasm around the tubes and mucous inside the tubes. This swelling makes it difficult to breathe. A sudden or severe asthma flare-up may be referred to as an asthma attack and will require asthma first aid.

According to Asthma Australia, it's often difficult to diagnose asthma in young children, especially as they can't perform the breathing tests as older children and adults to enable diagnosis of the condition. Your doctor or paediatrician will look at your child's symptoms and history and may give asthma medicine (such as Ventolin) to see what effect it has. A proper diagnosis of asthma takes time and children will usually have multiple wheezy episodes responsive to Ventolin before being given the diagnosis of asthma. It is important to remember that wheezing and coughing are very common in little children, even if they do not have asthma.

Prevention

Asthma cannot be prevented, but it can be well controlled. If possible, know what things trigger your child's asthma and try to avoid or reduce the incidences of these triggers. Some triggers cannot be avoided, so it is important to know how to manage the symptoms. Common triggers include:

+ Breathing infections such as colds and flu
+ Allergens such as dust mites and pollen
+ Exercise
+ Cigarette smoke

Sometimes even changes in the weather and emotions such as laughing or crying may trigger an asthma flare-up.

Another important way to help prevent and control flare-ups is to make sure your child is taking her medication properly. When you administer puffs of reliever medication, such as Ventolin, through a spacer (this is a tubular device that optimises the delivery of your child's inhaled asthma medication into her lungs), follow these steps:

+ Sit your child upright in a chair or in your lap.
+ Shake the medication puffer.
+ Ensure a good seal over your child's mouth and nose with the spacer mask.
+ Administer one puff of medication, followed by four breaths.
+ Repeat until you have given your child all the puffs prescribed.
+ If this does not help, call an ambulance on 000.
+ Follow DRSABCD if your child becomes unconscious (see **CPR**, pages 30–47).

Ensure you use a spacer, because it makes the delivery of the medicine so much more effective. Teenagers need particular encouragement, as it can be deemed uncool to be seen using one. While spacers come in different sizes, the Royal Children's Hospital in Melbourne recommends using small-volume spacers for children of all ages.

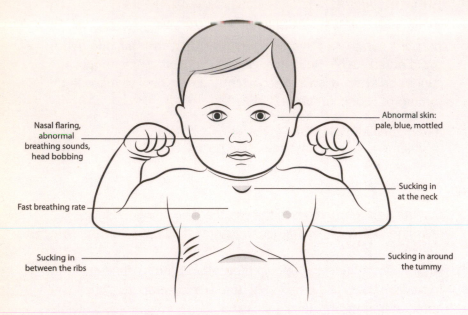

Nasal flaring, abnormal breathing sounds, head bobbing

Abnormal skin: pale, blue, mottled

Sucking in at the neck

Fast breathing rate

Sucking in between the ribs

Sucking in around the tummy

Possible signs of breathing difficulties during an asthma flare-up

Recognition

Symptoms of an asthma flare-up can vary depending on the severity. Asthma is also different for every child, so you need to get to know your child's symptoms and recognise when she is having a flare-up that is characteristic of her. It is important to know that you can't just rely on the sound of wheezing to tell you how severe your child's asthma is. She may not have a wheeze at all and be very sick, or have a loud wheeze and be okay. The illustration above shows possible signs and symptoms your child may show during an asthma flare-up. Remember, you know your child best, so get to know her symptoms.

Response

If your child is asthmatic, ensure your GP or paediatrician has provided you with an asthma action plan for her. Give this to your child's school or kindy and to other members of the family or people who regularly look after your child. Action plans are available for download from the Asthma Australia website (see **Resources**, pages 233–239).

In an emergency situation, a reliever medication (blue or grey puffer, usually Ventolin) should be used with a spacer. If you don't have a spacer available, improvise with a cardboard toilet roll or cup your hands over the child's nose and mouth.

First aid for an asthma attack is the **4 x 4 x 4 rule**:

Give four puffs of a reliever every four minutes, with four breaths on each puff.

+ Give four puffs, wait four minutes, give four more puffs, wait four minutes, give four more puffs.
+ If there is no relief, call an ambulance and continue giving four puffs every four minutes until help arrives.

Remember, always trust your instincts. If you are concerned for any reason, seek medical help.

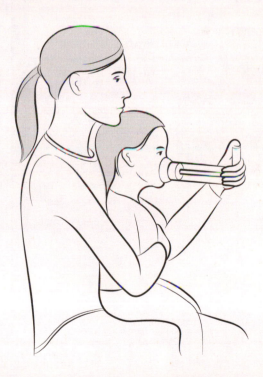

Using a spacer on a child

Kids' First Aid for Asthma

NationalAsthma CouncilAustralia
leading the attack against asthma

1 Sit the child upright.
Stay calm and reassure the child.
Don't leave the child alone.

2 Give 4 separate puffs of a reliever inhaler – blue/grey puffer (e.g. Ventolin, Asmol or Airomir)
Use a spacer, if available.
Give one puff at a time with 4–6 breaths after each puff.

Use the child's own reliever inhaler if available.
If not, use first aid kit reliever inhaler or borrow one.

OR

Give 2 separate doses of a Bricanyl inhaler
If a puffer is not available, you can use Bricanyl for **children aged 6 years and over**, even if the child does not normally use this.

3 Wait 4 minutes.
If the child still cannot breathe normally, **give 4 more puffs.**
Give one puff at a time (Use a spacer, if available).

Wait 4 minutes.
If the child still cannot breathe normally, **give 1 more dose.**

4 If the child still cannot breathe normally,
CALL AN AMBULANCE IMMEDIATELY (DIAL 000)
Say that a child is having an asthma attack.

Keep giving reliever.
Give 4 separate puffs every 4 minutes until the ambulance arrives.

If child still cannot breathe normally,
CALL AN AMBULANCE IMMEDIATELY (DIAL 000)
Say that a child is having an asthma attack.

Keep giving reliever
Give one dose every 4 minutes until the ambulance arrives.

HOW TO USE INHALER

WITH SPACER
Use spacer if available*

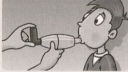

- Assemble spacer (attach mask if under 4)
- **Remove puffer cap and shake well**
- Insert puffer upright into spacer
- Place mouthpiece between child's teeth and seal lips around it OR place mask over child's mouth and nose forming a good seal
- **Press once firmly** on puffer to fire one puff into spacer
- **Child takes 4–6 breaths** in and out of spacer
- **Repeat** 1 puff at a time until 4 puffs taken – remember to shake the puffer before each puff
- Replace cap

If spacer not available for child under 7, cup child's/helper's hands around child's nose and mouth to form a good seal. Fire puffer through hands into air pocket. Follow steps for WITH SPACER.

WITHOUT SPACER
Kids over 7 if no spacer

- **Remove cap and shake well**
- Get child to **breathe out** away from puffer
- Place mouthpiece between child's teeth and seal lips around it
- Ask child to take slow deep breath
- **Press once firmly** on puffer while child breathes in
- Get child to hold breath for at least 4 seconds, then breathe out slowly away from puffer
- **Repeat** 1 puff at a time until 4 puffs taken – remember to shake the puffer before each puff
- Replace cap

BRICANYL
For children 6 and over only

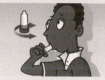

- Unscrew cover and remove
- **Hold inhaler upright and twist grip** around then back
- Get child to **breathe out** away from inhaler
- Place mouthpiece between child's teeth and seal lips around it
- Ask child to take a **big strong breath in**
- Ask child to breathe out slowly away from inhaler
- **Repeat** to take a second dose – remember to twist the grip both ways to reload before each dose
- Replace cover

Not Sure if it's Asthma?
CALL AMBULANCE IMMEDIATELY (DIAL 000)
If the child stays conscious and their main problem seems to be breathing, follow the asthma first aid steps. Asthma reliever medicine is unlikely to harm them even if they do not have asthma.

Severe Allergic Reactions
CALL AMBULANCE IMMEDIATELY (DIAL 000)
Follow the child's Action Plan for Anaphylaxis if available. If you know that the child has severe allergies and seems to be having a severe allergic reaction, use their adrenaline autoinjector (e.g. EpiPen, Anapen) before giving asthma reliever medicine.

Kids' first aid for Asthma
Courtesy of National Asthma Council Australia, 2016

SUMMARY

+ Asthma is a serious condition that can be managed with the correct treatment.
+ Understand your child's symptoms.
+ It's imperative to have an asthma action plan.
+ Follow the 4 x 4 x 4 rule in the event of an asthma attack.

Remember to remove the spacer lid!

When our son Jethro was four, he had asthma. It has mostly gone away since, but at the time we still sent him into preschool with an asthma pump and clear instructions on how to use it. One day, in the middle of the morning, I got a phone call from his preschool asking me to come in immediately. Jethro had been running around and his asthma had flared up. By the time I got there he had been given the pump but still looked a bit green, despite breathing without too much trouble. I assessed the situation. He didn't seem to be in any danger so I decided it would be best if I took him to the hospital rather than calling an ambulance.

When we arrived, he was given another pump by the staff and reacted well. I wondered why the first pump had not been so effective. It took us all a few weeks to realise that while we had taken the puffer lid off, we hadn't removed the spacer lid. He wasn't given any puffer at all by the school! We have since learned from our mistake and thrown away the spacer lid, as it is too easy to forget to remove it. Heavens alive, that could save a life.

Rosemary

BITES & STINGS

An English friend of mine once said to me that if anything bit her while she was in Australia, she would be hightailing it straight to the nearest hospital. She was convinced that every part of our native flora and fauna could kill her. Perhaps an extreme reaction, but she wasn't too far wrong! We do have a disproportionate number of the world's venomous creatures in Australia and it is wise to be familiar with what can hurt you and what is harmless. There is a lot of information out there on every creature, some of which I have listed in **Resources** (see pages 233–239).

When I think of bites, the first creatures that come to my mind are spiders and snakes. In reality, we are far more likely to be bitten by an insect, an animal such as a dog, or even another human!

As treatment varies depending on what has bitten you, the following first-aid advice is for the most common bites in Australia.

ANIMAL AND HUMAN BITES

Many preschoolers like to settle their disputes with a bite or two. Human bites are among the dirtiest you can get. Our mouths are awash with bacteria — remember this when your preschooler comes home with a set of teeth marks decorating her upper arm.

For animal bites, such as those from dogs, the first aid is the same as for human bites. Working as an emergency nurse, I have only seen a very small number of unprovoked animal bites. The overwhelming majority have happened when young kids were playing with animals. Many children just don't understand that getting right up close and personal with a dog or cat can be quite scary for the animal, or that picking them up for squeezy cuddles can make the animal think they are in mortal danger.

Being bitten is a tough way to learn to respect an animal's space, and hopefully it won't mean your child will become afraid of dogs — perhaps just more cautious. We've had a dog in our house since before the kids were born and he is an integral part of our family. I would never consider not having a dog or other pets around; teaching our kids how to respect and treat our animals is an important element of this.

Prevention

For dog bites, prevention is better than cure. As with Lucy, children under five are the most frequently affected, so teach your kids how to be gentle and interact appropriately with dogs and other household pets. Biting usually occurs when a child pulls a dog's tail or attempts to take a bone from a dog's mouth. And don't judge a dog by its size; those little balls of fluff can give quite a good nip.

School-aged children can be taught proper techniques to avoid a negative interaction with dogs. Cesar Milan, the world-renowned dog whisperer, recommends that you teach children the following:

+ Avoid approaching unfamiliar dogs.
+ Never scream at or run from a dog.
+ Never play with a dog without adult supervision.
+ Do not disturb a dog that is eating, sleeping or tending to puppies.
+ If a dog approaches, do not run away.
+ Always let a dog sniff you before patting it.

Recognition

Most bites from dogs occur to the face, neck and hands, and many human bites occur on the limbs. Without exception, any puncture wound from sharp, canine teeth should be examined by a doctor. Often they look okay on the outside but they can actually be quite deep, especially on the face. If your child is bitten on the face or hands, it's important to seek medical help. And remember to look for signs of infection. Redness and swelling of the bite area, pus on the wound, flu-like symptoms or fever can indicate infection, and medical help will be necessary.

Response

It takes quite a bit of force to break the skin's surface, so usually there is just some nasty bruising from a human bite (think: toddler fights over the Duplo). To treat bruising, a cold pack will do. However, if the skin is broken, you need to give it a very good clean with soap and water. Follow the recommended steps to control the bleeding (see **Bleeding**, pages 100–111), apply the antiseptic of your choice and cover the area with a dressing. If there is more than just a minor break in the skin, you should seek medical help. Deep or gaping wounds will need a proper washout and stitching in hospital. Cat scratches and bites can also be particularly nasty, so make sure you clean the area well with soap and water and treat as for human bites.

If a bite wound breaks the skin, it is important to make sure your child's immunisations are up to date, particularly tetanus and hepatitis immunisations. If you are overseas, make sure you seek medical treatment and know if rabies is an issue. There is specific treatment for your child if she is bitten in a particular geographical area where rabies is known to be present, so you need to seek urgent medical advice. And some general advice when travelling: *make sure you have travel insurance*!

INSECTS

BEES AND WASPS

Bee stings can be painful but the pain subsides quite quickly. However, this is not the case for severely allergic people, for whom a bee sting can be fatal. When a bee stings, it leaves behind the stinger with a sac of venom attached. In the past, the method to remove a bee sting was to scrape it to the side with your fingernail, a piece of stiff cardboard, a credit card or something similar, as the sting has barbs. This method was thought to be beneficial in avoiding squeezing the venom sac, which would inject more venom into the skin. Now there is evidence to show that it is more important to remove it quickly, rather than focus on the actual method of removal. So flick, scratch, wipe firmly, do whatever you can to get the sting out as soon as possible.

Prevention

Some species of bees and wasps aren't aggressive and only sting in self-defence. Others are cranky, but mostly because they think you are out to kill them, which may well be true. There are a few things you can do to minimise your chances of being stung. When it comes to kids, the main one is to teach them that if a bee or wasp is buzzing around, don't swat at it. This makes for an annoyed insect. Also, if your child is allergic to bee stings, don't dress her in a brightly coloured, floral patterned frock at a garden party because bees are attracted to bright colours.

If a bee gets caught in your clothing, stay calm. From personal experience, I would not recommend ripping your top off and jumping around in only your pants and bra at your daughter's dance school at pickup time. Not only does it make the bee very upset, it will also give your six-year-old an embarrassing story to tell everyone.

European wasp stings are also very common, and if a child or adult is stung repeatedly, an allergy can develop. It is very important to remove any European wasp nests from your backyard. They look like grey papier mâché, and you should leave their destruction to the professionals. Wasps love to hang around food and drink, particularly sweet drinks, so check before picking up that cup of juice or stick to water at a picnic.

Recognition

Bee and wasp stings are usually mild, with short-lived symptoms. They are more annoying than anything serious. Symptoms of a bee or wasp sting can include:

+ Sharp burning pain or itchiness at the site of the sting
+ A red welt and slight swelling around the site of the sting

Symptoms of a **mild reaction** usually go away in a few hours. Some kids have a bigger reaction to stings.

The signs and symptoms of a **moderate reaction** can include:

+ Extreme redness at and around the sting
+ Swelling at the site of the sting that continues to get bigger

Moderate reactions take longer to go away than mild reactions, sometimes a few days.

A **severe allergic reaction** to bee stings (anaphylaxis) can be life-threatening and require emergency medical care. Signs and symptoms may include:

+ Rash, possibly all over the body
+ Difficulty breathing
+ Swelling of the throat and tongue
+ Nausea and vomiting
+ Abdominal pain and diarrhoea
+ Dizziness
+ Floppiness
+ Loss of consciousness
+ Drop in blood pressure (shock)

Recognising when your child has these symptoms is very important because she will need *urgent medical help*.

Response

If your child is stung by a bee and has an anaphylactic reaction (life-threatening allergic reaction), remove the sting quickly —

ideally within seconds — and follow the first aid for anaphylaxis (see **Allergic Reaction & Anaphylaxis**, pages 62–67).

If your child is not anaphylactic to bee stings, follow these steps:

+ Remove the sting promptly.
+ Clean the affected area with soap and warm water.
+ Apply an ice pack or cold compress.

Seek medical help if there is a moderate to severe reaction. Your child may require medication to help with the symptoms. Always seek medical advice if you are concerned.

If your child is bitten by a European wasp:

+ Clean the affected area with soap and warm water.
+ Apply an ice pack or cold compress.
+ Give the child an analgesia such as paracetamol or ibuprofen.
+ Watch for anaphylaxis.
+ Seek medical help if there is excessive swelling at the site of the sting.

Kids and bees

When it comes to bees, the majority of kids are stung because they have unknowingly stood on one. When your child is in grass that contains flowers, always make sure she is wearing shoes. A swarm of bees, while aggressive in appearance, are usually very calm because they are searching for a place to live. They have no hive to protect, so there is no need to react obtrusively. If a swarm does land on your property, call a local bee club and they will have it removed safely.

However, if there is a hive of bees, make sure you do not let any family members near it. Whether they are feral or domestic, bees will protect their flight paths and sting anyone who comes near their hive.

Remember, bees do not want to hurt you or your children. If you keep a safe distance from them and make sure your child wears shoes in the grass, both parties should remain happy and safe.

Karen
Apiarist

MOSQUITOES

Mosquitoes are an annoying part of life, though usually not doing too much more harm other than inflicting a very itchy bite. Depending on where you live, however, they can also be carriers of blood-borne diseases such as Ross River virus, dengue fever and Murray Valley encephalitis. Fortunately, malaria is not so much of an issue in Australia. I was unlucky enough to contract malaria when my husband and I were volunteering in western Kenya. We were setting up medical camps with the locals, in a village right near Lake Victoria, a mosquito paradise. Luckily for me, I experienced only a mild case, as I was taking the preventive medication.

Prevention

Once a mosquito has finished its snack of human blood, it likes to lay its eggs in still water. Mosquito eggs hatch within 48 hours and the mosquitoes take five days to grow big enough to bite us.

During warm weather, regularly drain any standing water that has collected in plant pots, buckets, bird baths, inflatable pools, outdoor pet bowls and anywhere there is stagnant water where mosquito eggs can hatch. (Inflatable pools should be completely emptied after each use anyway, because of the drowning risk).

Mosquitoes also prefer dark colours, so putting your child in loose-fitting, light-coloured clothing can help prevent mosquito bites. There are lots of chemical repellents available; just be aware that some are quite toxic, especially for children. They should always be used sparingly, and make sure you read the label thoroughly. Natural alternatives designed especially for kids are available from good health-food shops and pharmacies. The strength of repellent needed is also dependent on where you live or where you are travelling to.

The Royal Children's Hospital Melbourne website, **www.rch.org.au**, has a helpful guide on insect repellent use in kids, specific to high- and low-risk areas. It recommends the following:

+ Read the entire label before use — look carefully at the level of DEET (diethyltoluamide) in the product.

+ Use the repellent only as directed by the manufacturer.
+ Roll-on preparations are preferable to sprays.
+ Apply sparingly to exposed skin.
+ For young children, insect repellents are safest if rubbed or sprayed on clothing rather than skin — never spray on the skin of children under one year old.
+ Do not apply to cuts, wounds or irritated skin.
+ Do not apply to areas around the eyes or mouth.
+ Do not apply to the lips, hands or fingers of young children.
+ When returning indoors, wash repellent off skin with soap and water.
+ Store repellents out of the reach of children, as ingestion may be harmful.

For more information on insect repellents and guidelines on the safe use of DEET in children, check out this link on the Royal Children's Hospital Melbourne website: **www.rch.org.au/kidsinfo/fact_sheets/Insect_repellents_ guidelines_for_safe_use/**

Recognition and Response

If your child has been bitten by mozzies, an itchy red lump may appear. Try not to let her scratch it (easier said than done), as this is a good way to make the bite infected and possibly leave a scar. Using anti-itch creams or other ointments such as thse containing papaw or aloe vera may help. Another good trick is to hold a cold pack on the bite for a minute or two. It will numb and soothe the area nicely. If your child is showing signs and symptoms of being unwell, if the bite site is swollen and looks infected, or if you are concerned for any other reason, seek medical help.

ANTS

Do you remember being bitten by a bull ant as a child? So very, very painful. Jack jumper ants, bull ants, jumping ants are all members of the *Myrmecia* genus, known for their feistiness and nasty sting. They're the species mostly responsible for the ant bites and stings we end up with. My favourite response to an ant sting comes from entomologist Justin Schmidt: 'Bold and unrelenting. Someone is using a power drill to excavate your ingrown toenail.'

If your child is bitten or stung by an ant, you will know about it very quickly. You can guarantee your child will be screaming the backyard down. Unless she has an allergy, you are just going to need to wash the area with soap and water, keep that cold pack on and put on her favourite TV show for distraction. Hang in there, but keep your eye out for a nasty reaction. The jack jumper ant is responsible for 90 per cent of the reactions in people who are anaphylactic to ant stings. (See **Anaphylaxis Action Plan** in Quick Reference colour section).

TICKS

Ticks are parasites that feed on animal and human blood. They are found all over Australia. There are many species of ticks and they can transmit viruses and bacteria when they bite. The most common one affecting humans is the paralysis tick, commonly known as a grass or bush tick. My six-year-old seems to pick up the little bloodsuckers every time we go bushwalking. Sometimes she doesn't even notice they are there; other times they have caused her immense pain at the bite site and a cracking headache. On our last camping trip, she ended up with two in her hair behind her right ear. After she named them Tiffany and Trevor, they were quickly removed. We do a full-body tick check regularly when we camp, but I missed those two in her hairline until she started complaining of a headache and scratching the area.

Prevention

Paralysis ticks are particularly common in bushy coastal areas along the eastern parts of Australia where it is moist and humid. Spring is the season when the adult ticks are most active, particularly after rain. They live in long grass and bushes, waiting for a nice warm snack to drop onto.

If you are going into a tick-infested area, the following steps may help prevent bites:

+ Dress your child in long-sleeved tops and long pants.
+ Tuck her pants into her socks so the ticks can't get under the pants.
+ Dress her in light-coloured clothing so it is easier to see the dark-coloured ticks.
+ Remove all clothing after visiting a tick-infested area and put it in a hot dryer for 20 minutes, or a hot wash, to kill any ticks.

Recognition

Ticks inject a toxin that may cause some redness and swelling at the bite site or a mild allergic reaction, but most tick bites cause few or no symptoms. If your child is allergic to tick bites, give prescribed medication and follow DRSABCD (see **CPR**, pages 30–47).

Tick paralysis, while uncommon, can pose a serious health threat. Some of the other serious tick-borne diseases occurring in Australia are Queensland tick typhus (also known as spotted fever) and Flinders Island spotted fever. Tick-induced mammalian meat allergy is a relatively new syndrome, in which people bitten by the paralysis tick can develop an anaphylactic reaction to eating meats and animal by-products such as gelatine.

Signs and symptoms of tick paralysis can include:

+ Rashes
+ Headache
+ Fever
+ Flu-like symptoms
+ Tenderness of the lymph nodes
+ Unsteadiness on feet
+ Sensitivity to bright light
+ Limb weakness
+ Paralysis of part of the face
+ A black scab at the bite site

If your child has any of these symptoms you must seek medical help.

Response

So, what is the best way to remove a tick? Previously, the advice was to gently pull the tick straight out with steady pressure, avoiding squeezing the body of the tick during removal. Now there is new evidence to show that this is not the best way.

Associate Professor Cheryl Van Nunen is a specialist in clinical immunology with Royal North Shore Hospital in Sydney and has published over 100 papers regarding stinging insects. Here's what she says:

'If it's a small tick, dab it, don't grab it. If it's a large tick, freeze it, don't squeeze it.'

This is great advice. When we remove ticks it is hard to avoid irritating them or squeezing their body, which causes them to inject more toxin and their allergenic saliva. The Australian Society of Clinical Immunology and Allergy (ASCIA) recommends the following technique to remove ticks:

For large ticks, freeze them off with an over-the-counter freezing spray such as WartOff. Your pharmacist can advise you on the best one to keep in your first-aid kit. When you freeze the tick, you stop it from injecting more toxin. Once frozen, the dead tick will drop off after a while, or you can use tweezers to remove it.

For smaller ticks (nymphs), dab a cream containing pyrethrum over the top. Once dead they will drop off. Avoid scratching them off.

Most importantly, don't let your child scratch. If you have difficulty or if there is still part of the tick in the skin, seek medical attention. If your child has a known tick allergy, follow your action plan.

Do not try to kill the tick with methylated spirits or any other chemicals. This will only cause the tick to inject more toxin and allergenic saliva.

Once the tick has been removed:

+ Wash the area with soap and water.
+ Seek medical help if part of the tick is left in the skin.
+ Seek medical help if your child shows any symptoms of tick diseases.

SNAKES AND SPIDERS

SNAKES AND FUNNEL-WEB SPIDERS

The reason I have grouped snakes and funnel-web spiders together is because they require the same first aid, and they are both dangerous!

Not all Australian snakes are venomous. There are around 100 venomous species of snake in Australia, and of these, only around a dozen are deadly. However, it is much better to be cautious and treat any snake as deadly. You wouldn't want to mistake a taipan for a children's python, and unless you are an expert, it can be very hard to distinguish between different snake species.

The Sydney funnel-web spider is also venomous and considered to be deadly to humans. The good news is that, according to scientists at the Australian Museum, there have not been any officially recorded deaths from a funnel-web spider bite since the introduction of antivenom in 1981.

If a spider has bitten your child, you are unsure what species it is and you are in an area where funnel-web spiders are around, err on the side of caution and apply a pressure bandage.

Prevention

Snakes are found in all parts of Australia and generally they just want to leave us alone. They are not usually aggressive, but if you stand on one it is going to get cranky and defend itself. Most bites occur when people try to catch or kill a snake.

Spiders also bite in self-defence, but it is an urban myth that funnel-web spiders jump and attack when biting. They do move rather quickly, though. The males are solitary and wander around looking for a mate. All recorded human deaths have been from the bite of the male.

Some tips to prevent bites in your family:

+ Wear closed-toed shoes and long pants, such as denim jeans, when bushwalking — no thongs or sandals, especially on the kids.
+ Teach your kids not to go poking their hands into fallen logs and thick scrub, under rocks or in other hiding places for snakes and spiders.
+ Teach your kids that snakes and spiders are not for petting.
+ Do the 'snake stomp' when walking through snake areas — walk with heavy footfalls to warn the snakes you are coming. Remember, they are scared of you.

As an emergency nurse, I treated a five-year-old girl who had been bitten by a small brown snake. She had picked it up thinking her brother had left his toy snake on the grass in the garden. Needless to say, the snake became very scared and bit her. She ran inside to her mum and told her she had been bitten, but her poor mum didn't believe her, as the little girl was prone to exaggeration and there was no sign of a bite on her. It is actually quite common to be bitten by a snake and see few or no marks, or even just a scratch. She very quickly became symptomatic. Luckily, her mum knew what to do and saved her life.

Recognition

As the five-year-old girl discovered, you won't always see a typical puncture wound when bitten by a snake or spider. Sometimes all it takes is a scratch from a fang to introduce venom beneath the skin. According to the experts at the University of Melbourne's Australian Venom Research Unit (AVRU), a snake can retain the biting reflex and its venom remains toxic for hours after its death.

Funnel-web spider fangs are rather large and you may well see puncture wounds at the bite site.

Signs of a funnel-web spider bite may include:

+ Visible puncture wounds
+ Pain at the bite site

+ Swelling and redness
+ Numbness in or around the mouth
+ Nausea and vomiting, and abdominal pain
+ Excessive saliva and sweating
+ Difficulty breathing
+ Drowsiness
+ Fast heart rate
+ Muscle spasms

Signs and symptoms of snakebite vary depending on the species of snake. Not all bites are painful: some only cause minor pain and a small amount of swelling to the bite site.

Symptoms can include *but are certainly not limited to*:

+ Puncture wounds at the bite site (not always visible)
+ Nausea and vomiting, and abdominal pain
+ Bleeding
+ Headache
+ Numbness
+ Fast heart rate
+ Difficulty breathing
+ Paralysis

Response

It is absolutely necessary to keep your child calm if she has been bitten by a snake or a funnel-web spider. As the AVRU states, keeping her calm is akin to 'stopping the clock' on the spread of venom.

It's very difficult to do, but it's also important that you stay calm in order to help her. If you are hysterical, your child will be too. It's as simple as that, so put your parent hat on, and think of your child's best interests.

Previously, the first-aid treatment for snakebite consisted of applying a tourniquet to cut off the blood supply. It is now understood that this is not effective and actually causes damage, as the venom is transferred into the lymph system. Today, we use the **pressure immobilisation technique (PIT)** to compress the limb and slow the flow of venom.

A pressure bandage is a wide, heavyweight bandage, such as one used to strap a sprained ankle. This should be wound over the site of the bite, all the way to the end of the limb (leaving the fingers or toes exposed), then all the way to the top of the limb, overlapping the bandage by half each time. The bandage should not be too tight. You should be able to stick one finger under the bandage, as you would apply a bandage to a sprained ankle — firm, but not enough to cut off the circulation. Splint the limb (see **Limb Injuries**, pages 160–169), try not to move your child and preferably get help to come to you.

1.

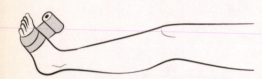

Starting at the bottom of the bitten limb,
wrap the pressure bandage upwards, leaving the toes or
fingers exposed

2.

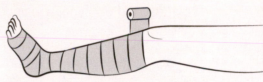

Overlap the bandage by a half each time,
as firmly as you would bandage
a sprained ankle

3.

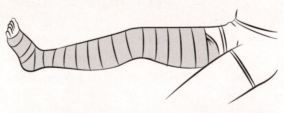

Continue to the top of the limb

Pressure immobilisation technique

The experts at the AVRU have compiled a list of DOs and DON'Ts when it comes to snake and funnel-web bites:

DOs:

+ DO follow DRSABCD (see **CPR**, pages 30–47).
+ DO retreat to a safe distance away from the snake.
+ DO calm the child, lay them down and keep them still.
+ DO remove rings, bracelets and any other constrictive objects from the bitten limb, so that if swelling occurs these do not cause an increased risk of serious harm due to restricted blood flow.
+ DO remain with the child at all times until help arrives. If you have no choice but to leave her in order to seek help, return as quickly as possible.
+ DO mark the bite site on the bandages if possible by using a pen to circle the area.

DON'Ts:

+ DO NOT try to catch, chase or kill the snake, as this may lead to another bite.
+ DO NOT give alcohol, tea, stimulants, food or medications without medical advice.
+ DO NOT wash the wound, apply hot or cold packs, cut the wound, use ligatures or tourniquets, or apply electric shocks, and do not suck the wound or use suction from any device.
+ DO NOT allow the child to walk or run.
+ DO NOT remove or loosen the pressure immobilisation bandages unless advised to do so by medical personnel.
+ DO NOT rely on traditional medicines or home remedies — obtain medical assistance urgently.

SUMMARY

To summarise, the AVRU suggests the following:

+ If others are present, have someone phone for medical assistance or go for help immediately.

+ Reassure your child and encourage her to remain calm and still.

+ As soon as possible, apply a broad pressure bandage, starting at the bite site, working towards the toes or fingers, then wrapping upward on the affected limb.

+ Leave the tips of the fingers or toes unbandaged to allow your child's circulation to be checked.

+ Do not remove her clothing, simply bandage over the top.

+ Bandage firmly as you would for a sprained ankle, but not so tightly that circulation is prevented.

+ Apply the bandage as far up the limb as possible to compress the lymphatic vessels.

+ It is vital to now apply a splint by binding a stick or suitable rigid item over the initial bandage.

+ Secure the splint to the bandaged limb by using another bandage. If you don't have another bandage, use clothing or something similar.

+ It is very important to keep the bitten limb (and your child) still.

+ Bind the splint firmly to as much of the limb as possible to prevent the child from moving her limb. This will also help restrict the spread of venom.

+ Seek urgent medical assistance now that first aid has been applied.

+ If your child becomes unconscious, follow DRSABCD (see **CPR**, pages 30–47) and keep going with compressions. Be aware that you may need to commence CPR.

> For more detailed information on snakes, spiders and other venomous creatures visit the AVRU's website, **www.avru.org.au**.

I heard an amazing survival story of a man who was repeatedly bitten by a brown snake in a sugar-cane plantation. The other workers who were with him were all trained in snakebite first aid, as it's a very real danger when working in plantations. A pressure bandage was applied, he was kept calm, and the air ambulance was called. It took two hours for the air ambulance to arrive, and by that time the man needed CPR. He was flown to a regional hospital with CPR going the entire time, given antivenom and put on life support. This very lucky man survived.

Staying calm, applying a pressure bandage and following DRSABCD are key.

REDBACKS AND OTHER SPIDERS

Redback spiders get quite a bad rap. In reality, it is highly unlikely that a redback spider will kill you. There have been no deaths recorded from redback spider envenomation since 1955 when the antivenom was introduced. However, their bites are very painful and are considered a medical emergency for children.

Prevention

Mature female redbacks are black with a red stripe on the back of their round abdomen. The stripe can vary in shape. Young females are smaller, usually brown with whitish markings. Male redback spiders are small and brown with red and white markings. The egg sacs look brown and woolly. Redback spider webs look quite untidy and are usually near the ground, with the spider hiding in a sheltered place nearby. Redback spiders are found in drier habitats throughout Australia, including built-up areas. They are commonly found in dry places around buildings, outdoor furniture, dog kennels, garden tools and plant pots. In the bush, redback spiders live under fallen tree branches and rocks. Clear debris away from around your house and yard, and discourage your kids from sticking their hands into spidery hidey places.

Recognition

Signs and symptoms of a redback spider bite may include:

+ Nausea
+ Vomiting
+ Abdominal or generalised pain
+ Sweating (especially around the bite site)
+ Restlessness
+ Palpitations
+ Weakness
+ Muscle spasm

Response

Antivenom is only given if the person bitten has strong symptoms. First aid for a redback spider bite does NOT include a pressure bandage, as it will only make the pain worse. As for snake and funnel-web spider bites, don't wash, cut or suck the bite area. Apply an ice pack to help with the pain, give analgesia (such as paracetamol or ibuprofen) and get medical help.

Other spider bites shouldn't cause more than some pain and perhaps some swelling at the bite site. White-tailed spiders are blamed for ulceration but scientific research shows that in the majority of cases the bites just cause redness and blistering. White-tailed spiders are one of the most common culprits when it comes to spider bites, as they don't live in webs but prefer to wander about and hang out in sheets, towels, shoes, wardrobes and so on. If your child is bitten by a white-tailed spider or other common spider (excluding the spiders mentioned earlier), apply ice to relieve the pain, give some paracetamol if necessary and seek medical help if you are concerned, or if the bite site is very red and/or swollen.

MARINE STINGS

Our waters are home to a variety of creatures that can bite or sting and it pays to be aware of them. Importantly, the first aid differs between creatures, so make sure you know what to do. The information provided in this section is from Dr Peter Fenner, also known as the Marine Medic, and from the AVRU. For more information visit www.marine-medic.com and www.avru.org.au.

BLUE-RINGED OCTOPUS

Prevention

Blue-ringed octopuses are rather pretty little brown creatures, around the size of an adult's thumb, with their tentacles curled up. Excitingly for children, they flash their little electric-blue rings when threatened. Not so excitingly, they are deadly. They like to hang out in rock pools around the coast of Australia, particularly in southern NSW and in Victoria. Kids love to go playing in rock pools, so just make sure there isn't one of these little nippers in there too.

I read a story in the paper recently about a little girl who collected shells at a popular Sydney beach. When she got home she decided her shells needed a wash and put them in the bath with her. Dad walked in to find a blue-ringed octopus floating in the bath! Needless to say, his daughter was pulled out very quickly. The octopus must have been hiding in one of the shells. Very. Lucky. Girl. Most blue-ringed octopus bites occur when one one of these creatures is picked up out of the water.

Recognition

The blue-ringed octopus gives a relatively painless bite with its beak. However, very rapidly after being bitten, your child's lips and tongue may become numb. With serious bites, your child's breathing will become affected very quickly. Breathing difficulty develops, and without treatment, breathing can stop altogether.

Response

Treatment is the same as for a snake and funnel-web spider bite (see pages 87–89, 90):

+ Apply a pressure bandage.
+ Follow DRSABCD (see **CPR**, pages 30–47).
+ Call for an ambulance on 000.

JELLYFISH

There are many different types of jellyfish that live in our waters. Some do no harm; others are deadly. It pays to know what types hang out in the waters you and your children are swimming in.

Prevention

The majority of harmful jellyfish live in the warmer tropical waters. Dangerous species include box and Irukandji jellyfish. Stinger season typically starts in November and runs through to March.

The experts in the Marine Stingers Group, formed by Surf Life Saving Australia and the Queensland Government, recommend the following precautions when swimming:

+ Always swim at patrolled beaches and between the red and yellow flags.
+ Look for and obey safety signs.
+ Don't enter the water when the beach is closed.
+ Ask a lifesaver or lifeguard for help and advice if you need it.
+ Don't touch marine stingers washed up on the beach, as they can still sting you.

In **tropical waters**, it is also recommended you take these additional measures:

+ Swim within the stinger nets where provided.
+ Wear a full-body lycra suit, or equivalent, to provide a good measure of protection against marine stings, particularly during stinger season.
+ Enter the water slowly — this gives marine stingers time to move away.

Recognition

Depending on the type of jellyfish, signs and symptoms of a sting can differ. Box jellyfish stings can result in tentacle marks, severe pain, breathing difficulties and eventual collapse, whereas Irukandji jellyfish stings are usually small with a raised red area (welt), and symptoms occur around 20 to 40 minutes after the sting. These symptoms may include severe back pain and headache, nausea and vomiting, profuse sweating, agitation, and a feeling of panic or 'impending doom'. The symptoms for the different types of marine stingers are included in the table on pages 96–99.

Response

If a jellyfish stings your child in **tropical waters**, apply the following first aid:

+ Follow DRSABCD (see **CPR**, pages 30–47).
+ Remove any remaining tentacles with your fingers, but do not rub the sting site.
+ Pour vinegar over the sting site for at least 30 seconds.
+ If no vinegar is available, pick off the tentacles and rinse with seawater, not fresh water.
+ Ensure medical help is on the way.

In **non-tropical waters**, the bluebottle is the main culprit for many painful stings. Our friends at Surf Life Saving Australia (**sls.com.au**) recommend hot water to relieve the pain of bluebottle stings. Vinegar is not recommended. If you child has been stung by a bluebottle:

+ Keep her calm.
+ Don't let her rub the affected area.
+ Pick off any remaining tentacles with your fingers (a harmless prickling may be felt).
+ Rinse the stung area well with seawater to remove any invisible stinging cells.
+ Place her affected body part in the hottest water she can comfortably tolerate (test it yourself first).
+ If the heat does not relieve the pain, or if hot water is not available, apply cold packs or wrapped ice cubes.
+ Do not wash the sting with fresh water.

The following recognition and response table has been created with information from both the Marine Medic and AVRU websites.

Creature	Possible signs and symptoms	Pressure immobilisation technique?	First aid	Where do I seek help?
Bees and wasps	Redness, pain and swelling at sting site	No	Remove sting promptly (bee) Wash with soap and water Apply cold pack	Moderate reaction: see your GP Severe reaction: follow action plan Call ambulance 000
Mosquitoes	Redness, minor swelling and itch at bite site	No	Apply cold pack	Excessive swelling or signs of infection: see your GP
Ants	Redness, intense pain and minor swelling to sting site	No	Wash with soap and water Apply cold pack	Severe allergic reaction: follow action plan Call ambulance 000
Ticks	Redness, minor swelling, irritation at site	No	Remove with freezing spray (adult tick) or pyrethrum cream (nymph)	Severe allergic reaction: follow action plan Call ambulance 000
Funnel-web spider	Pain, tingling lips, twitching tongue, drooling, headache, nausea, vomiting, abdominal pain, sweating, breathing difficulties, seizures and collapse	Yes	Apply pressure bandage and immobilise the entire bitten limb Keep the victim calm and still DRSABCD	Call ambulance 000

Creature	Possible signs and symptoms	Pressure immobilisation technique?	First aid	Where do I seek help?
Redback spider	Sweating (including around bite site), nausea, abdominal or chest pain, general unwellness	No	Apply cold pack	Seek medical help if the victim is a young child or more than a mild reaction occurs
Other spiders (including white-tailed spiders)	Mild pain at bite site, mild redness and swelling	No	Wash area with soap and water Apply cold pack	See your GP if more than a mild local reaction occurs
Snakes (including sea snakes)	Headache, nausea and vomiting, abdominal pain, muscle weakness or paralysis, difficulty breathing or swallowing, blurry vision, collapse (the bite site may not always be visible)	Yes	Apply pressure bandage and immobilise the entire bitten limb Keep the victim calm and still DRSABCD	Call ambulance 000
Irukandji jellyfish	Sting site is usually small with a raised red area (welt) 20–40 minutes after the sting: severe back pain and headache, nausea vomiting, profuse sweating, agitation, a feeling of panic or 'impending doom'	No	Wash sting site with copious amounts of vinegar (use seawater if vinegar is not available) Pick off remaining tentacles Apply cold pack DRSABCD	Call ambulance 000

Creature	Possible signs and symptoms	Pressure immobilisation technique?	First aid	Where do I seek help?
Box jellyfish	Tentacle marks, severe pain, breathing difficulties, collapse	No	Wash sting site with copious amounts of vinegar (use seawater if vinegar is not available) Pick off remaining tentacles Apply cold pack DRSABCD	Call ambulance 000
Other tropical jellyfish	Mild to severe pain, tentacle marks, rash, redness, blistering and swelling to sting site	No	Wash sting site with copious amounts of vinegar (use seawater if vinegar is not available) Pick off remaining tentacles Apply cold pack	Seek assistance from a lifeguard if available Seek medical assistance, call ambulance 000 if severe reaction
Bluebottle (non-tropical)	Mild to severe pain, tentacle marks, rash, redness, blistering and swelling to sting site	No	Wash sting site with copious amounts of seawater Pick off tentacles Place in hot water (not so hot as to cause burns) for 20 minutes at a time for 2 hours	Severe pain, difficulty breathing or stung on the face, throat, or large sting area: Call ambulance 000
Cone snails (Cone shells)	Pain, swelling to site, numbness, muscle weakness, breathing difficulties	Yes	Apply pressure bandage and immobilise the entire bitten limb Keep the victim calm and still DRSABCD	Call ambulance 000

Creature	Possible signs and symptoms	Pressure immobilisation technique?	First aid	Where do I seek help?
Blue-ringed octopus	Little or no pain, tingling around mouth, mild weakness, breathing difficulties	Yes	Apply pressure bandage and immobilise the entire bitten limb Keep the victim calm and still DRSABCD	Call ambulance 000
Stonefish and other fish	Severe pain, swelling and tenderness to sting site, skin discolouration (blue), dizziness, nausea and vomiting, abdominal pain, breathing difficulties, collapse	No	Wash sting site with copious amounts of **fresh** water Place in hot water (be cautious – not so hot as to cause burns) for 20 minutes at a time for 2 hours Apply antiseptic to wound. DRSABCD	Seek medical help Severe reaction: Call ambulance 000

Sources: www.marine-medic.com.au, www.avru.org.au

If your child has a known allergy to any of these creatures, always follow your action plan and if necessary seek urgent medical help.

BLEEDING

Cuts and grazes. There isn't a child who will escape her youth without one, some or many of these injuries. They are a childhood rite of passage. From tumbles off scooters to fingers slammed in doors, you need to know how to treat the wound and stay calm while doing it. Many people hate the sight of blood, but as I've already mentioned, when it comes to your children you have to keep yourself together. Children look to adults when they are sick or injured. If we freak out, they will too. Like many adults, many kids hate the sight of blood, so I always recommend keeping a red-coloured hand towel in your first-aid kit. It helps disguise the blood, keeping those squeamish tummies more settled. This works particularly well for kids with special needs such as autism and other sensory issues.

Prevention

Parenting is about a lot of things, but a big slice of it is about using your common sense, especially around kids, because frankly, they often don't have much of their own. If your child rides a bike, scooter, skateboard or anything else that needs wheels or involves speed, using proper safety equipment such as a helmet and knee and elbow pads is *mandatory*.

For very young children especially, little fingers and slamming doors are not a good combination, so door bumpers are a good investment. When kids get a bit older, it's important to teach them how to handle kitchen knives safely. My nurse friend Glenda puts it beautifully:

> ## Reduce the risk
>
> *Have you have ever wondered about the little things you could do around the house to keep your child safe as she grows?*
>
> *One suggestion is to decommission all coffee tables until after your child reaches school age. Coffee tables seem to be the perfect height for toddlers to cruise, climb and explore — there is a natural attraction! However, you should know that coffee tables are frequently implicated in a variety of toddler injuries. They include eyebrow, forehead, scalp and chin cuts, lip lacerations and dental injuries, burns from hot drinks and foods, falls, and choking on or swallowing small hazardous items such as coins — even the odd alcoholic drink. Reduce the risk and make supervision easier.'*
>
> **Glenda**
> Paediatric nurse practitioner

Recognition

So how do you know if your child's cut needs stitches, and how much blood is too much when it comes to nosebleeds? Fortunately most wounds in kids are minor and can be dealt with at home.

Look at the wound. Is it gaping? Can you see deeply into it? Is there fatty tissue, muscle or bone? Are the edges jagged or unable to come together easily? Is it in a tricky area such as around the lip, eye or ear? If the answer to any of these questions is yes, it's likely your child will need some stitches or skin glue. However, don't give her anything to eat or drink before going to your nearest hospital or GP in case she needs to have surgery, or even some nitrous oxide (laughing gas) to make the experience a little more bearable.

If the bleeding doesn't stop after first-aid treatment, or if a wound is showing signs of infection, you'll also need to seek medical help. Trust your instincts. If you think a doctor needs to see the wound, they probably do.

If you notice that the blood is spurting, apply very firm pressure and call an ambulance on 000. It is likely to be an artery that has been damaged, and this is a medical emergency. This is also the reason why you should never pull anything out of a deep wound. Small intrusions such as minor splinters need to be dug out, but anything deep must be kept in place. Stabilise the wound, apply indirect pressure and seek medical attention.

Infection is always a risk with any wound. Signs and symptoms of infection include:

+ Redness and/or swelling around the wound
+ Pus coming from the wound
+ Flu-like symptoms
+ Fever
+ Excessive pain
+ The body part affected is hot to touch compared with other parts of the body

You need to get medical help if your child has any of these symptoms, as antibiotics may be needed.

There are some wounds that need medical attention even if they do stop bleeding easily: cuts that go through the border of the lip, cuts to the cartilage of the ear, deep puncture wounds and very dirty cuts that you can't clean or that might have something inside such as broken glass. If you are not sure what to do, err on the side of caution and seek medical help.

LACERATIONS (CUTS)

Lacerations are defined as tears in body tissue such as skin from a blow, impact or other injury. Small children are very cleverly designed to withstand impact. However, kids do tend to be prone to lacerations, and the most common places for these are above the forehead and below the chin — the main points of impact.

It is usually the force of the blow that causes the skin to split, and the blood flow from even a small head wound is usually substantial. On many occasions, I have seen a child come into the emergency department holding a blood-soaked tea towel over a wound for dear life, frightened that the body part they were pressing onto might fall off if they let go. Then after some cajoling and/or bribery, the nurse has removed the tea towel only to find that the cut was less than a centimetre long.

Response

In first aid, the key response to bleeding is to stop it, and the best way to stop a wound from bleeding is by applying firm, direct pressure over the top for a minimum of five minutes. For the parents of a bleeding, screaming toddler, this can feel like two hours. Apply pressure using any material that is clean and dry. If your first aid kit isn't handy, a tea towel or face washer is perfect. Out at the park (and let's face it, accidents usually happen when you're out and about), use a scarf, the child's jumper or T-shirt, or even a pair of socks. Apply very firm pressure over the wound.

If the wound is minor, after applying pressure for five minutes, clean it with some saline or water, ensuring all the dirt is out of the wound, and apply the antiseptic of your choice. Then cover the wound if you need to. Remember, common sense is key. If you are concerned about the wound, seek medical help.

Using Steri-Strips or 'butterfly' Band-Aids can be very useful. Most kids love having Band-Aids applied, so keep plenty in stock.

If the wound has something embedded in it, such as a stick or a pair of scissors do not pull the object out. You need to apply pressure around the object to stop the bleeding (otherwise known as indirect pressure).

One of my many little 'Superman' friends, Jacob, once injured himself falling out of a tree and onto a branch below. A stick the size of a ballpoint pen went into the back of his leg. His parents knew first aid and understood that they should not pull the stick out. Rather, the better option was to stabilise it, apply pressure and get help.

Jacob's parents wrapped two tea towels around the base of the stick and applied a bandage to keep it in place. This stopped the stick from wobbling around and also applied pressure around the wound to stop it bleeding. They couldn't put Jacob into his car seat to take him to the hospital, so they called an ambulance. Jacob

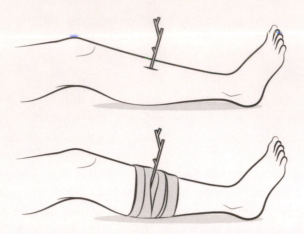

Bandaging a wound that has an embedded object

needed surgery to remove the stick, and was very lucky his parents did not pull it out, as it had severed one of the major blood vessels behind his knee. The stick had been acting as a plug.

Jacob would not have bled to death in seconds if they had pulled the stick out or anything as dramatic as that. But doing so could have caused more damage to the leg and he would have suffered significant blood loss.

SUMMARY

+ Apply firm direct pressure over the wound using clean and dry material.
+ Keep pressure on for five minutes.
+ If blood is spurting from the wound, apply firm, direct pressure and call 000.
+ Don't pull out anything that could be deeply embedded in a wound — stabilise it and seek medical help.
+ If the wound is gaping, dirty, deep or in a tricky area such as around the lip, eye or ear, seek medical help.
+ Don't give your child anything to eat or drink until she is seen by a doctor.
+ If the wound is minor, clean it, apply an antiseptic of your choice if necessary and cover with a bandage.

A pea in his forehead

About a month before the birth of our second child, my husband and I were having dinner with a few friends one evening. Our toddler son and his little playmate (the son of two of our friends) were set up in a room upstairs full of toys. It was their favourite place and they played there often. The safety gate was in the doorway and the room was safe (or so we all thought). As we ate, we could hear lots of happy laughter and innocent noises — until there was one loud crash!

We all raced upstairs to discover the kids had found a packet of dried peas meant for the garden, and had scattered them all over the floor. Our son, Jake, had then climbed up onto the bed (which none of us had thought he was able to do), had managed to get over the high end of bed and had fallen onto the wooden floor. He had fallen head-first onto one of the dried peas on the floor and it was embedded in his forehead. There was no blood, but there was no way the pea was coming out. We took him to the emergency department, where it was surgically removed. Apparently, it went down as the most unusual accident they had ever dealt with. The medical staff told us that the best we'd done was to leave it there, because Jake's forehead would have seriously bled if we had tried to remove it.

Jake is now a colorectal surgeon and the baby I was pregnant with is an ear, nose and throat surgeon. Jake still has a very minor mark on his head from the embedded pea but otherwise no long-term damage.

Jenny

ABRASIONS (GRAZES)

Grazes are one injury almost every child is guaranteed to have at some point. Kids come off skateboards, bikes, scooters — basically anything that can move will attract a child. They climb on it, fall off it and lose some skin in the process. Even though grazes are usually minor, they can be very painful and occasionally quite dirty. If you are concerned, seek medical help.

Response

First, the dirt needs to be removed. One of the best ways to do this is to put your child in a warm bath. Wash out the dirt using a soft flannel. Unfortunately, you need to be a mean parent and make sure the wound is clean, even though they will be protesting. You don't want the wound to end up infected. Much better to have a few minutes of yelling and a nice clean wound than an infected one. Don't scrub too hard; this can cause more trauma to the wound and a whole lot of pain, not to mention noise. A bit of chat about an upcoming birthday wish list while you're gently agitating the muck out should do the trick.

Pat the wound dry with something that doesn't shed fibres — you don't want fluff sticking to the graze. Try to apply an antiseptic of your choice; wounds heal better in a moist environment. However, getting a toddler to leave a dressing in place can be quite tricky. Applying a wound-healing gel or something like pawpaw cream over the graze before applying a non-stick dressing will promote healing. Just remember the dressing will need to be changed if it gets wet. If you have a child who will not tolerate a dressing, watch out for of things like clothes and sheets that might stick to the graze while it dries out.

As the graze heals, it will become itchy. Kids will then pick at the scab, which can cause scarring and further bleeding. They need to be encouraged to leave it alone.

SUMMARY

+ Wash the wound with water and remove dirt.
+ Apply an antiseptic of your choice and a non-stick dressing if needed.
+ Look for signs of infection.
+ Seek medical help if you are concerned.

AMPUTATIONS AND CRUSH INJURIES

Little fingers are very curious, and this can often lead to injuries. Crushed fingers in doors are a common injury in young children. Door hinges in your home exert a great deal of pressure, more than enough to crush or amputate the tip of a child's finger. Car doors are also a popular place for kids to get their fingers caught.

Response

If your child crushes her finger, your priority is to stop the bleeding. You need to apply firm, direct pressure to the finger with something clean and dry. Ideally this should be sterile gauze out of your first-aid kit, but anything clean and dry will do. Call an ambulance on 000. You will then need to look at the finger. Don't panic if a part of the finger has been amputated — modern medicine can work wonders!

Once the bleeding is under control, you will need to collect the part that has been amputated, if this is what has happened. Do not put the amputated part straight onto ice or into water, as this will cause more damage and reduce the part's viability for reattachment. Instead, wrap it in some damp (NOT wet) sterile gauze and seal it in a plastic bag. A zip-lock sandwich bag is ideal. If you don't have any sterile gauze, paper towel is a good option; just make sure whatever you place it in is not wet, just either damp or dry. If the amputated part is very dirty, gently rinse it under some running tap water first. Place the sealed bag on an ice slurry. (A slurry is water mixed with ice.) A good way of doing this is to put water and ice in a plastic container, cup or another zip-lock bag, then put the sealed bag with the amputated part into the container, cup or bag.

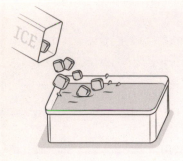

Create a slurry (ice and water)

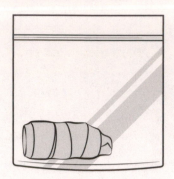

Place the body part in a zip-lock bag

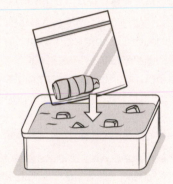

Put the sealed bag into the slurry

Preserving an amputated body part

Saving an amputated body part

It is vital that the amputated part remain with the injured child. I have heard lots of stories of how people have become separated from their body parts in transit to the hospital.

Children who have a crush injury or an amputation usually need to have an operation, not just to repair the wound, but also for a thorough washout to prevent infection. I am constantly amazed by the plastic surgeons and what they can successfully reattach, so even if you are unsure about whether it is worth bringing the amputated part, bring it anyway, just in case.

> ## SUMMARY
>
> + The priority is to apply firm, direct pressure to stop or slow the bleeding.
> + Call an ambulance on 000.
> + If there is an amputated part, recover it and rinse it gently under tap water if dirty.
> + Place the part in damp (NOT wet) gauze or paper towel and seal in a plastic bag.
> + Place the bag on an ice slurry.
> + Do not put the part directly in ice or water.
> + The amputated part should remain with the injured child.

NOSEBLEEDS

Nosebleeds can be very common in children and it can look like they have lost a fair amount of blood. However, nosebleeds often look much worse than they actually are. They are common and can usually be managed at home. They can be caused by knocks to the head or nose, picking the nose, inserting objects up the nose, dry air, allergies or infection. The bleeding happens when the fragile blood vessels in the nose burst.

Response

If your child has a nosebleed, keep her calm. Crying increases pressure in the nose and will make the bleeding worse. Get her to lean forward and pinch her nostrils (the soft part below the bridge of the nose) with firm pressure. Ask her to breathe through her mouth. Apply a cold pack or cold face washer to the bridge of her nose (if she will tolerate it). Keep applying the cold pack with pressure for 10 minutes.

Don't be tempted to keep checking whether the bleed has stopped, just keep the pressure on for the full 10 minutes. This is where it's handy to have a timer in your first-aid kit, or you can use the timer on your phone. If the bleeding hasn't stopped after 10 minutes, repeat for another 10.

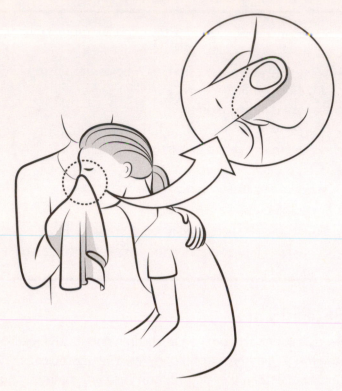

First aid for nosebleeds

Once the bleeding stops, it is very important to stop your child from sniffing or blowing her nose for at least 15 minutes. This is a hard thing to do, as clots in the nose feel awful. You also need to stop her from picking. Your child may vomit blood after a nosebleed if the blood has been running down the back of her throat and she has swallowed it. Don't worry, this is normal.

If her nose does not stop bleeding, or if the nosebleeds are frequent, seek medical help. If your child has a bleeding disorder always follow the action plan from your paediatrician or GP.

SUMMARY

+ Keep your child calm.
+ Lean her forward.
+ Pinch her nostrils and ask her to breathe through her mouth.
+ Place a cold pack or face washer over the bridge of her nose.
+ Apply pressure for 10 minutes.
+ Ask your child not to sniff, pick at or blow her nose for at least 15 minutes.
+ Seek medical help if the bleeding does not stop.
+ If your child has a bleeding disorder always follow the action plan from your paediatrician or GP.

BURNS

Ice? Butter? Egg white? At one time or another, these foods (and some others) have all been suggested as the best first-aid treatment for burns in both adults and children. But are they effective? The research says no. Burns are defined as injury to tissues caused by contact with heat, flame, chemicals, electricity or radiation, and are one of the leading causes of injury in children, especially toddlers. According to the World Health Organization (**www.who.int/mediacentre/factsheets/fs365/en**), 260 children from around the world die from a burn injury every day.

TYPES OF BURNS

Prevention is key when it comes to burns, but first we need to understand the types of burns that may injure a child.

Thermal burns

A thermal burn is a burn from contact with heat. Hot water, cups of tea, soup and other liquids, hot objects such as heaters and hair straighteners as well as the obvious flame burns are just a few of the common causes of thermal burns.

Sadly, scalds from hot liquids are very common, with scalds in children under five accounting for over 65 per cent of burns.
An inquisitive, thirsty toddler being taught to drink from a cup will reach for a drink, regardless of the temperature of the contents.

It is *critical* for you to be aware of this. Apart from the obvious causes of scalds, such as hot drinks, pulling the handles of saucepans off the stove, hot water from the bath and so on, be aware of other sources. Don't drink hot drinks with babies in your arms. I have seen children in carry pouches have hot coffee splashed on their heads when the lid on the takeaway coffee has fallen off. Be aware.

Electrical burns

Electrical burns can occur if your child comes into contact with electricity. If your child is injured by such a burn, first make sure that you do not place yourself in danger — switch off the circuit breaker (safety switch) before touching her, so that you do not become a victim too! Be prepared to follow DRSABCD (see **CPR**, pages 30–47) as electrical injuries can cause damage to the heart and other organs, not just burns to the skin. Be aware that your child may have two burns — where the electrical current both entered and exited her body.

Chemical burns

A chemical burn occurs when there is contact with a chemical irritant (an acid or an alkaline chemical). Common chemical burns are inflicted by household cleaners such as bleach or drain cleaner as well as the very dangerous lithium ion (button) batteries.

Radiation burns

For kids, the most common cause of radiation burn is sunburn.

Friction burns

The easiest friction burns to think about for kids are carpet burn and the too-frequent treadmill burn. See **www.kidshealth.schn. health.nsw.gov.au/burns-prevention** for information on burns and treadmills — they're a thing!

PREVENTING AND TREATING BURNS

Prevention

When it comes to preventing burns, a good approach is to put yourself in your child's shoes (not literally) and get down to her level. What can she reach? That coffee table top that was too high for her before may now be well within reach, allowing her to pull herself up to view what's there. Or maybe your curious toddler wants to help cook and can now reach the stovetop? It pays to think about this kind of thing regularly when you have little ones in the house. Remember, they grow and develop so quickly.

As always, prevention is better than cure. You need to teach your child that hot equals danger. Kids also learn by experience. If it's happened once, even toddlers can understand that if they touch the hot oven door again, it will hurt.

Flame burns such as those from campfires, candles and matches are also a source of serious injury in children. Remember to use the STOP, DROP, COVER, ROLL technique:

+ STOP straight away.
+ DROP quickly to the ground.
+ COVER your face with your hands, elbows tucked in.
+ ROLL over and over on the ground to put the flames out.

Hot liquid scalds

To prevent scalds from occurring around the home:

+ Turn stovetop saucepan handles in towards the wall.
+ Use a child-proof stove guard.
+ Keep hot drinks out of reach.
+ If you carry your baby in a pouch, don't drink your hot coffee above her head.
+ Keep vaporisers out of reach.

Babies and children's skin burns at much lower temperatures than that of adults. A good way to minimise scalds is to turn your hot-water system down to 50 degrees Celsius. Most hot water systems are set at around 70 degrees Celsius. It only takes a second to burn a child with water at this temperature.

Other thermal burns

+ Keep hair dryers and straighteners out of reach of small fingers.
+ Keep electrical appliance cords out of reach (don't let them dangle down for little hands to grab).
+ Use fireplace or heater guards.
+ Make sure the campfire is fully out before you leave camp (douse with water, not dirt or sand).

Chemical burns

+ Keep all household chemicals out of reach.
+ Make sure button batteries are kept out of reach, and devices containing these batteries are secure (see **Foreign Bodies**, pages 149–152).

Sunburn

+ Keep to the shade in the hottest parts of the day.
+ Cover up — dress your child (in particular, your baby) in long sleeves and long pants.
+ Apply sunscreen to all exposed skin.
+ Keep that hat on (easier said than done with a wilful toddler).
+ Download the **Sunsmart** app.

When it comes to little babies, many parents cover up the pram with a blanket when it is sleep time, or to protect them from the sun. Caution needs to be used here. Because prams are not designed to have a full covering (apart from the mesh type, often provided with your pram when you purchase it), you need to make sure there is plenty of air ventilation. Dr Svante Norgren, a paediatrician at the Astrid Lindgren Children's Hospital in Stockholm, suggests a pram can trap heat like a thermos. One experiment showed that the temperature inside a covered pram was 12 degrees Celsius higher than outside the pram. Imagine that on a 30-degree day!

Recognition

Burns used to be described in degrees — first, second and third. This has now changed.

They now are described as superficial (affecting only the superficial layers of skin), partial-thickness (affecting down to the underlying layers of the skin) and full-thickness (affecting all layers of the skin). It may not be possible to see how deep the burn is until a few days after the incident. Partial-thickness burns in particular are extremely painful. Full-thickness burns may not hurt, as the nerve endings are so badly damaged.

Response

The most important part of first aid for burns is to cool the affected area with cold running tap water for a minimum of 20 minutes.

Yes, 20 minutes seems an incredibly long time, especially with a toddler, but it's exactly what you need to do. It is imperative that you get water onto the burn as soon as possible, as it will not only help with the pain but it will also help to stop further damage from occurring to the skin. Even if there is no water available straight away, you should cool the burn with water as soon as it is available. You can apply cool water up to three hours after the burn injury and it will still be effective.

Of course, we are not always near running tap water when a burn occurs. You may need to improvise. Do you have a bottle of water? Is there a tap anywhere around? An irrigation system? I know of a child who burned his leg from the exhaust of the motorbike he was riding on an outback property. His dad put him in a nearby dam, soaked the boy's jumper in the water and kept it on the burn until they reached the house, where his dad then put him in the shower. If you do put your child's burned area into a sink or bowl of water, it is very important to change the water regularly, as it will quickly heat up and become ineffective.

Running water helps the healing process, but don't let your child get cold. Only cool the burned areas, and keep the other areas warm.

I recall two-year-old Molly, who pulled a freshly brewed cup of tea off the kitchen bench and onto herself. Her mum immediately removed Molly's clothes, put her under the shower, and called an ambulance. Luckily, Molly's mum also removed her nappy. Nappies soak up the hot water and retain heat, which can create genital burns. *Always remove the nappy!*

Give your child some pain relief, such as paracetamol. The hospital or ambulance will also give your child some pain relief medication. The Centre for Children's Burns and Trauma Research, based at the Royal Children's Hospital in Brisbane, recommends a four-step approach to the first-aid treatment of burns – REMOVE, COOL, COVER, SEEK:

+ Quickly REMOVE any clothing and jewellery from the burned area. This is important, because jewellery and clothing can trap heat on her skin and restrict blood flow to the area if it starts to swell. However, if your child's clothes are stuck to her skin, do not remove them, and do not pop any blisters.
+ Immediately COOL the area with running water (such as from a cold tap) for a minimum of 20 minutes. During this time, only apply the water to the burned area. Keep your child warm with a blanket, or by holding her so that only the burned area is under the water and your body heat is keeping the rest of her warm.
+ Use cling wrap, a clean cloth or a non-stick dressing to COVER and protect the burned area after cooling. Do not use ice, creams, oil or other substances. They will not help the wound to heal and they may cause infection or more damage. They will also interfere with the doctor's examination.
+ Seek medical attention for ALL children's burns: call 000 for major burns; go to a hospital or your GP for minor burns. For adults, if the burn is larger than a 50-cent coin, or is on the face, hands or groin area, or is white in colour (which means it is deep), seek medical attention.

Electrical burns

Always make sure you are safe before you touch the patient. Turn off the electricity using a wooden object or the safety switch so that you are not electrocuted or burned as well. Then REMOVE, COOL, COVER, SEEK.

Chemical burns

Use a cloth to brush any chemicals off the skin — do not use your bare hands. Then REMOVE, COOL, COVER, SEEK.

Sunburn

If the sunburn is extensive, put your child in a cool shower. Otherwise, cool the affected area with cold water for 20 minutes. If the sunburn covers a large area or is in delicate areas, or if your child feels unwell, seek medical attention. Babies with sunburn need to be reviewed medically as they can become quite unwell (they can lose vital fluids through the burn). Remember, with sunburn, prevention is better than cure.

SUMMARY

+ For flame burns: STOP, DROP, COVER, ROLL.

+ Remove clothing (including your child's nappy), unless it is stuck to the skin.

+ Cool the burn with cool running tap water for a minimum of 20 minutes.

+ Cover the burn with cling wrap, a clean cloth or a non-stick dressing.

+ Seek medical help.

+ You can apply first aid for up to three hours after the burn, and it will still be effective.

Hot coffee burn: 'I knew it was really bad'

On the day of my daughter Billie's christening, we were about 10 minutes away from leaving for the church. I decided I'd better have a coffee, as I hadn't had a chance for one that morning. I made a cup and sat it on my bedside table while I put my shoes on. In that split second, Billie, who at the time wasn't walking but pulling herself up, did just that on the bedside table, and in the process picked up the cup and tipped it over her chin and neck, and down over her chest and torso. It was a full mug of black coffee, so basically, boiling water. I grabbed her immediately and, in our clothes, we both jumped into a cold shower.

At the time, my husband was at the party venue setting up the balloons, so it was only my non English speaking grandparents from interstate and my 13-year-old goddaughter at home with us. They all came rushing in and it was very traumatic. I took Billie's top off while under the water and the skin was peeling before my eyes. I knew it was really bad. My goddaughter brought me the phone and I called an ambulance. The ambulance arrived and we got out of the shower. By this time, we had been in there for about 15 minutes. Billie was very cold. They raced us, sirens blazing, to our nearest children's hospital. At this stage, the fear was that she might have consumed some of the boiling water and that her throat could have been burned, affecting her airways.

On arrival, we were swamped by doctors, and later that evening we were transferred to another paediatric hospital after it was decided the burns covered approximately 10 per cent of her body and she needed specialist treatment. The burn site was cleaned and properly dressed, which again was very traumatic.

We were there for a few nights, and a week later, Billie had skin-graft surgery on her torso. When the doctors brought her out to Recovery, they told us that once they had her in theatre and were able to clean the area again, they could see a lot of healing had occurred under the dead skin. So they'd only performed two minor skin grafts. Billie now wears compression clothes and will do so for another six months. There will be scarring, but it will hopefully be very minor by time she reaches adulthood.

Many doctors at the hospital, including the surgeon, asked me how it was that I got her in the water so quickly. The truth is, I have no idea. I've had no first-aid training and it was just a natural, immediate reaction for me. They've told me time and time again that getting Billie into the shower made the difference between a couple of small skin grafts and what would have been deep, deep burns and multiple skin-graft surgeries.

Georgia

Cool running water was the key

Our son Jack was 22 months old and we were staying in a holiday house with visiting family. It had been a ragged few days, as torrential rain had left us all housebound — four adults and four active kids.

Very early on the Sunday morning, my sister-in-law made two cups of tea and put them on the table in the living room. Before any of us could think, Jack walked over and pulled one of the cups onto himself, the hot tea pouring down his chest, luckily missing his face. His blood-curdling scream jolted us into action. I grabbed Jack and pulled off his pyjama top and nappy, gave him to my husband Ant, and got them into the coolest shower possible. Jack's skin was 'bubbling' and his screaming was heartbreaking. While Ant and Jack were in the shower I got my brother-in-law to call 000 and direct the ambulance. It was an agonising wait.

After 15 minutes, Jack stopped screaming and went very quiet, which was probably even worse than the screaming. The ambulance arrived and asked how long he'd been under the shower. As it was just under 20 minutes, they kept him there until we'd passed the 20-minute mark. They gave Jack morphine for the pain and then loaded the three of us into the ambulance.

At the hospital Jack was treated and photos of his burns were sent to the burns unit at a major hospital in Brisbane, where we lived. A couple of days later, when we were back home, we took him to the burns unit and they patched his chest with special silver gauze that had two small pipes for us to inject water into twice daily to keep the wound moist. The first patch stayed on for seven days and the second for five days. Once the patches were off, we were instructed to put sorbolene cream on at every nappy change.

Today, Jack is six. There is no visible scarring on his tummy, and when we ask him, he has no memory of the accident. Thank goodness I'd heard of a similar story and knew to put his burns under cool running water for 20 minutes — that was key.

Petrina

CHOKING

As a general rule, kids and babies can choke on anything that's smaller than a D-size battery. This means a lot of everyday objects are fair game for a would-be choking incident. In our CPR Kids classes, the number one question we are asked is what to do if a child chokes, and there is always at least one person who has had first-hand experience of this. Choking occurs when a person's airway (windpipe or trachea) is partially or completely blocked. This blockage makes breathing a rather critical problem.

As mentioned, babies and toddlers learn by exploring their world. One of the ways they do this (often to the angst of their parents) is by putting everything they come across into their mouths. This is completely normal, and an important part of their development, but when they get their hands on the wrong objects, choking can be an issue.

In my paediatric emergency nursing career, I have seen lots of children who have had choking episodes. Luckily, the majority come in on the ambulance stretcher breathing well, with Mum and Dad in tears because the child has choked at home and turned blue. First aid has been given and the object has come flying out, but the shock of seeing their child choking has been all too real. It is imperative that you know what to do.

Prevention

When it comes to preventing choking in kids, there are four key things you need to know:

1. Chop up the grapes (and sausages too)

A child's airway is smaller than an adult's. This makes children more likely to get objects stuck in their throats. A grape is the perfect size to lodge in a child's airway, and is incredibly difficult to get out once stuck. Always chop up grapes and cherry tomatoes into quarters when giving them to your little one, or just squish them with your fingers. As long as they are no longer circular they are unlikely to get stuck. This goes for any food you offer your child — carrots, cucumbers, sausages (chop into batons, not discs) and so on.

2. Sit down to eat

Good luck with this if you have a toddler. You need the skills of a highly trained negotiator to keep a toddler at the table. Letting them run around with food in their mouths, however, does pose a risk that they will inhale the contents. Make it a rule in your house that when eating, your little one must be sitting on her bottom. Your child will be more likely to stay put if you are sitting there too, so use the time during the meal to talk and connect — a great habit to get into, especially as they get older.

3. Keep them in your sights

Even though it may be tempting to have a quick shower or get something done in another room while your child is occupied with eating (and strapped into the high chair to prevent escape), stay with them. Choking can be silent, so always remain where you can see them.

4. Keep the little things out of reach

Small items, such as Lego, button batteries, marbles, anything smaller than a D-size battery, are choking hazards for a child. Keep little items out of reach and ensure toys are age-appropriate and in good condition. Broken toys can have small parts that break off and become a hazard. Older siblings need to be encouraged to keep their smaller toys away from the little ones. Button batteries (see **Foreign Bodies**, pages 149–152) are lethal if swallowed. Not only do they pose a choking risk, but they will also cause severe burns. Keep them out of reach, and seek IMMEDIATE emergency help if you think your child has swallowed one.

Recognition

Babies often gag when they start to eat solids. Gagging is different from choking. The gag reflex is what causes your baby to thrust her tongue forward whenever the back of her throat is stimulated. This could simply be a reaction to having something in her mouth (or it might just be your cooking!). Stand back!

The gagging reflex in babies can be quite sensitive until they get used to swallowing food. They may cough and turn red, but will usually clear the offending piece of food quickly and continue eating. Remember, gagging is normal.

As I explain earlier, choking happens when the airway is either partially or completely blocked. If it's partially blocked, your baby will start to cough to clear it, which is usually very effective. If the airway is completely blocked, your baby may not be making any sound and will be unable to cough effectively. This is when you need to intervene very quickly with **back blows** and **chest thrusts** (see pages 126–127).

Older children tend to choke when they're running around while eating or sucking on lollipops, pens, toys — you name it. One little stumble and down the hatch it goes.

If your child or baby has what we call an **effective cough**, don't intervene; let her clear it herself. An effective cough means that a child is able to take a big breath of air in and then emit a strong, forceful cough out. This is the body's reflex, or defence mechanism. The idea is to expel the air from the lungs at high speed to pop out the offending object or piece of food. It is very tempting in this situation to whack a child on the back, however if you whack her while she is taking a big breath in, the object might dislodge and go further down, potentially obstructing the airway completely.

An object can often get lodged in the oesophagus (food pipe) too. This is a medical emergency. Symptoms include an inability to swallow and excessive drooling.

I recently saw a six-year-old who had been running with a dollar coin in her mouth and stumbled (she said she didn't have a pocket to put it in). Down her throat it went. It lodged in her oesophagus, very close to the entrance to her airway. She was able to talk but couldn't swallow her saliva, so she was drooling copious amounts of it. She quickly went to the operating theatre to have it removed under a general anaesthetic. Let's hope she doesn't substitute her mouth for a pocket anymore.

Babies and children **look very scared** when they are choking and are unable to cough effectively. They may also be **silent**. You can see the fear in their eyes. This is one of the important differences between a child who is gagging and one who is choking. The gagging child doesn't look scared — they might turn red and cough, but they settle down again very quickly. A child with an obstructed airway will not settle.

A choking child or baby may show the following signs:

Baby

+ Irritable
+ Distressed and clingy
+ Drooling excessively
+ Hoarse or not crying
+ Silent, unable to breathe
+ Red then blue in the face
+ Coughing persistently
+ Breathing noisily or with difficulty

Child

+ Holding her neck (universal sign)
+ Distressed
+ Irritable, panicked
+ Drooling excessively
+ Red then blue in the face

+ Coughing persistently
+ Unable to talk
+ Breathing noisily or with difficulty
+ Silent, unable to breathe

Trust me, you will know if your child is choking. Every parent I have spoken to whose child has had a serious choking episode has said it was unmistakeable.

Response

Often people think the Heimlich manoeuvre is the way to go for a choking child, but I urge you to resist the temptation. Just don't do it. In a young child it can cause damage to the internal organs, so stick to back blows and chest thrusts, as discussed next.

Babies can gag on milk, particularly if the flow is too fast. Often if you are breastfeeding and you have a fast letdown, your baby can get too much too quickly, causing her to pull off the breast. Sometimes babies can go quite red and cough for a period of time, but usually they stop quickly and the hardest task is to calm them down and get them latched on again. They can also be mucousy if they have a cold. You don't usually need to intervene, just sit your baby upright, leaning forward slightly or hold her face-down, supporting her jaw. Remember, milk is liquid and will clear with coughing. If it is mucous and it isn't clearing, you may need to give some gentle back blows and chest thrusts (described on pages 126–127).

First aid for choking differs depending on your baby or child's symptoms:

1. Unconscious patient
2. Conscious patient with an effective cough
3. Conscious patient with an ineffective cough, or silent

1. Unconscious patient

If your baby or child is unconscious, call an ambulance on 000 and follow DRSABCD (see **CPR**, pages 30–47). You need to remove the food or object from her mouth, but ONLY if you can grasp it easily. If you put your fingers down her throat (finger sweep), there is a very real danger of pushing the food or object further down, so only try to get it out if you can easily grasp it. Finger sweeps are not recommended in babies for this reason.

2. Conscious patient with an effective cough

As I described earlier, an effective cough is when a baby or child is able to take a big breath in and forcefully cough out. The idea is that the forceful cough will pop the object out.

Remember, if a baby or child has an effective cough, no matter how tempting it is to whack her on the back, don't do it. If you hit her on the back while she is taking a big breath in you might dislodge it while she is taking that big breath and she will then inhale it further, potentially causing more of an obstruction.

Stay with your child, comfort her and encourage her to keep coughing. She will probably vomit, and this is okay. Watch your child like a hawk, though, because if her cough becomes ineffective, you need to intervene with back blows very quickly.

3. Conscious patient with an ineffective cough, or silent

This is very scary, both for the choking baby or child and the parent. If your child or baby is not able to cough forcefully, or she is silent (even scarier), you need to intervene very quickly.

If your baby is conscious with an ineffective cough, pick her up and place her tummy down along your leg, while supporting her jaw. Having her pointing down uses gravity to assist you. Pull your arm back and give her a forceful blow between her shoulder blades. This is called a **back blow**. The idea of the back blow is not just to whack her on the back, but also to push the air forcefully out and pop out the food or object. Give up to five back blows. If the object comes out, there is no need to give all five blows.

If this does not work, turn your baby over onto her back. While supporting her head, push down with two or three fingers in the middle of her breastbone in line with the nipples (same place as CPR — see **CPR**, pages 30–47) in a thrusting motion. This is called a **chest thrust**. A chest thrust is sharp and deliberate, whereas CPR is smooth and rhythmical.

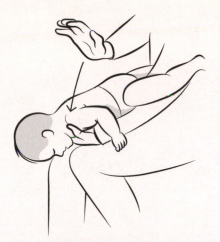

Back blows on a baby

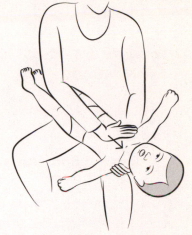

Chest thrusts on a baby

Give up to five chest thrusts. If this does not work, go back to five back blows and continue to alternate until the obstruction is cleared; your baby will probably vomit too. If your baby becomes unconscious before the obstruction is cleared, follow DRSABCD (see **CPR**, pages 30–47).

The same procedure should be followed for children. If your child is too heavy to place down along your leg, stand her up and tilt her forward. You will need to brace an older child with your arm for the back blows and support them for chest thrusts. Hopefully, the movement up and down will help to dislodge the object.

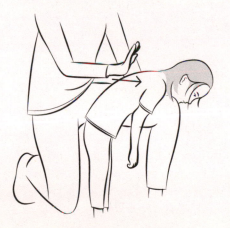

Back blows on a child

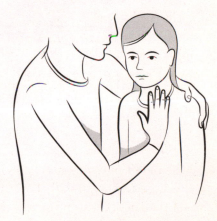

Chest thrusts on a child

Foreign Body Airway Obstruction (Choking)

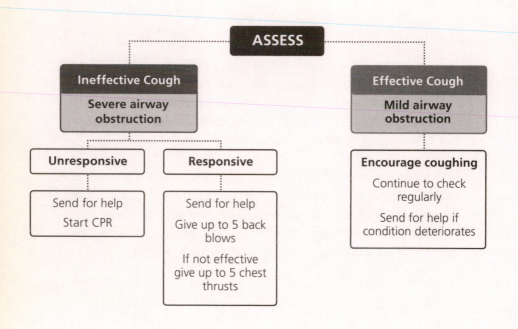

What to do when the airway is obstructed by a foreign object
Chart courtesy of Australian and New Zealand Committee
on Resuscitation (ANZCOR)

Choking: 'we knew what we had to do'

Our son Luca had a choking episode recently and we had to do back blows. It was so scary, but thanks to the first-aid course we had recently attended, we knew what we had to do. We only had to do two blows and out popped the biscuit piece. It probably would have eventually gone soft and crumbled anyway, but Luca definitely wasn't breathing and was quite distressed. We thanked our lucky stars that we had made the effort to do a first-aid course, as we were able to deal with the situation as best we could ... and then have a glass of wine once we put him to bed!

I think just having attended the course made me feel more confident — I still totally panicked on the inside, but I knew what I had to do on the outside. I have recommended doing a first-aid course to all my friends because I truly think it saved us from a very bad situation.

Kristy (& Chris)

'He almost choked on a marble'

When my son Jason was nearly two, he almost choked on a marble. I noticed him playing with the marbles on the lounge-room floor and immediately went to clean them up, but just when I thought I'd got them all, I looked up to see him standing in front of me, not saying anything. It was pretty clear something was wrong. He looked surprised. His lips were turning a bluish colour and his mouth was slightly parted.

I realised quite quickly that he was choking and pulled him over my knee. I tilted him head-down and patted his back hard at least four or five times. The last few pats were hard enough to dislodge the marble and it popped out and went sailing across the lounge-room floor. Jason made a gasping sound and cried afterwards. After lots of cuddles we put the marbles away in a safe place, out of reach.

I was relieved that I'd known what to do and had been able to help my son — otherwise the situation could have been a whole lot worse.

Ian

'First aid for choking is simple but so effective'

As a children's emergency nurse, I have seen many children brought into hospital following a choking incident. Fortunately, due to the effectiveness of first aid in relieving choking, the majority of these children get to go home. I had never had to perform back blows or chest thrusts on a choking child until my own son began choking at home. It was a moment that I will never forget.

My eight-month-old son was in the kitchen with his dad, having his dinner. He was strapped into his high chair eating a variety of finger foods while my husband was entertaining him. I was in the lounge Skyping my parents and could hear them laughing together. My son finds my husband hilarious and he was belly-laughing and squealing with excitement. The next moment my husband screamed at me in a voice I had never heard him use before, and which turned my blood to ice: 'Laura, he's not breathing.'

I raced into the kitchen to see my son sitting silent, open-mouthed and wide-eyed, still strapped into his high chair, turning blue around the lips. Instinct took over, and before I knew what I was doing, I had yanked him out of his chair and was holding him head-down.

I smacked him hard on his back between his shoulder blades.

One back blow: nothing.

Another back blow: still nothing.

Third back blow and the offending piece of avocado shot out of his mouth. He took a large intake of breath and then vomited everywhere.

I burst into tears. My husband cried too. It was such a huge relief. My son was looking at both of us, completely bewildered and wondering what all the fuss was about.

Feeding avocado to my child was something that had never worried me. Yet he'd managed to inhale it when he was laughing and it had stopped him from breathing. We later noticed he had a bruise on his back where I had performed the back blows, but otherwise he appeared completely unaffected by the whole incident. It could have been a very different story, and I dread even to imagine what the alternative could have been. I am so grateful that I knew what to do.

First aid for choking is simple but so effective and, literally, life-saving.

Laura
Children's emergency nurse

DENTAL INJURIES

It seems that teeth can cause trouble across the age spectrum, from painful eruptions in teething babies to dental injuries in permanent adult teeth. It is estimated that up to 50 per cent of children will have some type of injury to a tooth before they reach adulthood.

Every baby is different. Some get their teeth early; others don't get teeth until they are 12 months old. Usually a child will have a full set of 20 teeth by around the age of three years. Around the age of six years the permanent teeth begin to come through; my seven-year-old is still waiting for her first visit from the Tooth Fairy. By the time we are 21 we should have between 28 and 32 teeth, depending on whether we have wisdom teeth, otherwise known as the third molars.

We need to ensure that we care for and protect those precious little choppers.

Prevention

We know we need to look after our children's teeth by ensuring our children brush and floss at least twice a day. Regular check-ups at the dentist are also important. Even so, we all know accidents happen, so it's just as important to know what to do if a tooth gets injured or knocked out. According to paediatric dentists Dr Dennis McTigue and Dr Amy Thompson, falls, sports-related injuries and fights are the most common causes of tooth injury in children.

Mouth injuries can also occur when a child trips or is pushed with an object in her mouth. Your first-aid treatment might not only help your child, but also save you an expensive dentist bill.

When playing sport, mouthguards are the number-one priority for preventing dental injuries. It is much cheaper to buy a mouthguard than to pay for the dental bills if an injury happens. But it's also important to stop toddlers from running around with sippy cups or other objects in their mouths. If they fall, you can almost guarantee a mouth or dental injury.

Recognition

As a parent, you can often be at a loss as to what to do if your child has a dental injury. Dr McTigue and Dr Thompson advise taking your child to the emergency dentist or emergency department if:

+ There is pain, tenderness or sensitivity (to heat, cold or pressure) in a tooth.
+ There is a broken, loose or missing tooth after trauma (the tooth could have been inhaled through the nose or swallowed).
+ There is bleeding that does not stop after you have applied pressure for 10 minutes.
+ There is pain in the jaw when your child opens or closes her mouth.
+ Your child is having difficulty swallowing or breathing.
+ Your child develops a fever or other signs of infection after a mouth or tooth injury.
+ You are concerned about your child's condition for any other reason.

When my daughter was two years old she slipped as she was climbing out of the bath ('No, Mummy, *I* do it!'). There was a sickening thud as she face-planted right into the side of the bath. There was blood everywhere; her bottom teeth had gone straight through the skin just below her bottom lip. Her tiny baby teeth were impacted into her gum. We took her to the hospital and fortunately her teeth didn't need to be removed. Today, all she has to show for her bath-exiting independence is a small scar just below her lip. Phew!

Response

Deciduous teeth (usually known as baby teeth) start falling out around the age of seven. If your child injures a baby tooth, the first-aid treatment is different from the treatment for injury to or loss of a permanent tooth.

Baby (deciduous) teeth

If your child knocks out a baby tooth, do not put it back into the socket. Doing this can cause damage to the permanent teeth that have not yet come down (or up). Instead, get your child to bite down onto a face washer or clean cloth to help stop the bleeding. Put the tooth or tooth fragments into milk or saliva (see below) and go to your dentist or an emergency dental service. You will need to make a dental visit urgently if the tooth is impacted into the gum.

If there is no emergency dental service in your area, take your child to your nearest hospital's emergency department. (See **Resources**, pages 233–239.)

Permanent teeth

If your child has knocked out a permanent tooth, stay calm and pick up the tooth by the crown (the part that you usually see in the mouth). DO NOT touch the root. If the tooth has visible dirt on it, rinse it in milk, saliva or saline for a few seconds. Do not rub or scrub it. If possible, put it back into the socket and get your child to bite down onto a face washer or clean cloth to keep the tooth in place. If you are unable to put the tooth back into the socket, put it in milk or saliva. A zip-lock bag is perfect for this. If you are out at the park or in another place where no milk or bag is available, put the tooth into your mouth between your cheek and gums. This will keep it moist and safe. If your child is older, she can pop it into her own mouth, between her cheek and gums. Obviously, this is not advisable for younger children, as it is likely they will swallow the tooth.

Seek immediate help from your dentist or an emergency dental service.

SUMMARY

For injury to or loss of a **deciduous (baby) tooth**:

+ Stay calm.
+ Pick up the tooth by the crown (top).
+ DO NOT touch the root.
+ Get your child to bite down on a washer or clean cloth.
+ Put the tooth in milk or saliva, not water.
+ DO NOT put the tooth back into the socket.
+ Go to your dentist or an emergency dental service.

For injury to or loss of a **permanent tooth**:

+ Stay calm.
+ Pick up the tooth by the crown (top).
+ DO NOT touch the root.
+ Rinse gently in milk, saliva or saline if the root is dirty; do not scrub or wash in water.
+ Place the tooth back into the socket if possible.
+ Get your child to bite down on a washer or clean cloth.
+ Put the tooth in milk, saline solution or saliva if you cannot put it back into the socket.
+ Seek urgent dental help.

Common dental injuries

As an orthodontist, the most common dental injury I see in kids is teeth that have been knocked out or chipped. These injuries are usually first seen by a dentist or attended to in an emergency department, and then if specific treatment is required, the patients are referred to me. I also see facial injuries, such as when an impact to the mouth has caused the gum to be pulled from the bone — if this happens to your child, go straight to your nearest emergency department or call an ambulance. It's a serious injury, usually accompanied by plenty of blood, and it needs specialist medical treatment.

If your child chips or loses a deciduous (baby) tooth, just hang on to it so your dentist can confirm it hasn't been inhaled or ingested. It's also good for your dentist to make sure there are no remaining pieces of the tooth left in your child's mouth, in case the tooth is broken and/or has only partially been knocked out.

If your child loses a permanent tooth, you should seek help from your dentist within a couple of hours if possible. The sooner you get the child and tooth to the dentist, the better the chance the tooth has of 'taking' after being reimplanted. An easy way to preserve the tooth is to spit into a plastic bag and place the tooth in the saliva. Do not rinse the tooth in water, as this will compromise the cells growing in the root of the tooth.

If your child is calm enough, ask her to gently bite down using a small cloth to cushion the area and absorb blood. If the tooth is dirty before you rinse it, make sure you tell your dentist and arrange for your child to have a tetanus injection.

If your child is a little older and has braces, this can often (but not always) save your child's teeth from being knocked out. Often the injury looks a lot worse than it is, since the metal on the braces may well cut her lips and cheeks. You should see your orthodontist as soon as possible after any trauma to your child's mouth. Any cuts or ulcers from braces should be treated with medication from your orthodontist — unfortunately, this is part of wearing braces and these minor irritations usually clear up within a few days.

If your kids play a contact sport such as rugby league, rugby union, soccer, hockey or AFL, wearing a mouthguard is absolutely mandatory. For sports such as basketball, touch football and netball, I also highly recommend it. In some countries, kids wear mouthguards skateboarding and bike riding.

Get a mouthguard fitted by your dentist, especially if your child has braces. The boil-and-bite mouthguards are better than wearing nothing, but I liken it to buying a pair of school shoes: have them properly fitted and your child's feet will be properly protected. Check the mouthguard at the beginning of each season until teeth are fully grown. Quite simply, my message about mouthguards is this: spend a little, save a lot.

Dr Jason Yee
Orthodontist

DROWNING

A child can drown in as little as five centimetres of water, in less than 30 seconds. You should never forget this fact.

> Drowning is the biggest cause of death in Australian children aged five and under, but is usually preventable. Alarmingly, up to 70 per cent of drowning deaths can be attributed to lack of adult supervision (www.watersafety.vic.gov.au).

When it comes to drowning, most of us automatically think of pools. In Australia, water and pool safety is drummed into us from an early age. It is part of our culture. We know to fence our pools, watch our kids in the water and send them to swimming lessons. But tragedies still happen. I have seen children who have drowned in pools, but I have seen more toddlers who have drowned in baths. According to Kidsafe Victoria, the home is the most common environment for a toddler to drown. Families have been irreparably damaged by these preventable accidents.

Prevention

When your baby is young, it is easy to lift her out of the bath, dry her off and put her into her pyjamas. Once she's settled, you go back to the bath to get the toys out and drain the water. There is no danger that your baby will go back into the water-filled bath, because she is not yet mobile. Once she does become mobile, however, leaving the water in the bath is a huge danger.

Think of the times you've taken your child out of the bath to get her dressed and you've been distracted by a ringing phone, dinner preparations or the requests of other siblings. Now think about your little one wandering back into the bathroom, hopping into the (enticing) toy-filled bath and silently slipping under the water.

This is a preventable tragedy. Make it a rule in your home: **baby out, plug out**. Never leave water in the bath.

Nappy buckets, backyard ponds, inflatable kiddy pools, outdoor bins, creeks, rivers and dams are also risky places for kids. Kidsafe Victoria has a valuable online resource to help you assess the water risks around your home. It only takes a few minutes, and it can potentially save a life.

Do the water safety audit at **www.kidsafevic.com.au/wsa**.

Tips for water safety and kids

+ As soon as your children have finished splashing in their inflatable pool, tip out the water and store the pool upright so more water cannot collect in it.
+ At parties or gatherings where there is a pool, allocate an adult to watch over the kids and swap every 10 minutes. Drowning deaths have occurred with lots of people around because everyone thought that someone else was watching the kids in the pool. Make the allocated person wear a special hat or scarf or another identifying object, and pass it on to the next watcher when their shift is over.
+ Always pull the plug out of the bath as soon as you've finished bathing the kids.
+ Keep lids on nappy buckets or keep them out of reach of children.
+ Put mesh or fencing over backyard ponds or water features.
+ Teach your kids to swim and make sure the whole family is aware of water safety.

+ Ensure your pool's fencing meets Australian Standards and check it regularly — make sure you are compliant with the laws. Make sure your pool is registered with your local council (see **Resources**, pages 233–239).
+ Keep furniture and pot plants away from pool fencing so children can't climb over them to access the pool.
+ If you're boating, ensure any children on board wear life jackets at all times.
+ Teach your child to swim between the flags at the beach — don't rely on lifeguards to watch her.
+ Dams are the most common place for drowning on farms, so restrict your child's play area so she does not have access to water.
+ Never ever take your eyes off your small child in water and stay within arm's reach.

Recognition

In the movies and on TV, drowning is always portrayed as a loud, splashing event with lots of screaming and cries for help. This couldn't be further from the truth. When a person gets out of depth in the water and starts to panic, there might be some arm-waving and splashing but the actual drowning can be silent. A child can fall or slip into the water and may be unable to get back up to the surface, or be face-down in the water. People have drowned with other swimmers only metres away, as they looked calm and not in any danger.

A drowning person may:

+ Be unable to shout or wave for help.
+ Have their head low in the water with their mouth at water level.
+ Have their head tilted back with their mouth open.
+ Have their eyes open and be looking fearful.
+ Be hyperventilating or gasping.
+ Be trying to swim, or have their arms and legs moving but be unable to go anywhere.
+ Be trying to float on their back.

On a recent trip to the beach with my family, we were paddling at knee depth in a beach lagoon. There was a sharp drop-off and the bottom of the lagoon became quite deep, so I was concentrating on watching my girls closely. Not too far from us was a group of boys playing rugby in the water, and about 20 metres away from the boys, a woman floating on a boogie board with her daughter on the woman's back. But there was something about this woman and her daughter that just wasn't quite right. The water was very deep and all of a sudden the woman's head slipped under the water, and the boogie board floated away.

My husband is trained in water rescue and dived straight in. He swam to her just as she slipped under the water again, with her daughter still fearfully clinging to her back. He managed to grab hold of them both and brought them the short distance to shore. There was lots of coughing, but mother and daughter, although exhausted and very shaken, were both okay. They were tourists who couldn't swim and thought they would be safe if they took a boogie board to float on. Even though the beach was packed and the boys had been playing only metres away, no one had noticed this woman was drowning. She simply had her head low in the water.

Drowning is silent. I hope the woman and her daughter won't make that mistake ever again.

Response

You must follow DRSABCD (see **CPR**, pages 30–47) when rescuing a baby or child from water. Importantly, make sure *you* are safe before you attempt to rescue a child. You need to ensure you are not going to become a victim too. A drowning child is usually in a state of panic or exhaustion, or both, and may inadvertently pull you under in her terror. Unless you are trained in water rescue, it is recommended that you throw a rope or another object to pull her in.

You then need to commence DRSABCD quickly. Only roll the child onto her side if she has foreign matter (such as vomit) obstructing her airway. Promptly roll her back as soon as the airway is clear and continue DRSABCD.

It is imperative that there are minimal interruptions to compressions. Continue with compressions and breaths at a rate of 30:2 even if the child has frothy or clear liquid coming out of her mouth. Only turn her onto her side to clear the airway if there is debris or vomit.

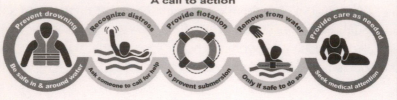

Courtesy of the International Life Saving Federation

The Drowning Chain of Survival from the International Life Saving Federation summarises the steps to prevent and survive drowning:

+ **Prevent drowning** — take appropriate steps to be safe in and around water.

+ **Recognise distress** — know the signs to look for and if necessary call for help.

+ **Provide flotation** — to keep the person afloat.

+ **Remove from water** — only if safe to do so.

+ **Provide care as needed** — commence DRSABCD and call an ambulance on 000.

SUMMARY

+ Prevention is better than cure — always think of water safety.

+ Apply Basic Life Support following DRSABCD.

'My child was drowning but no one knew'

It was July, and my four-year-old was having a week of swimming lessons at our local pool during the school holidays. Although he was confident in the water, due to enforced periods of time spent out of the water, he lacked some basic skills and was far behind his peers in ability.

It was the last day of lessons and his swimming ability had improved greatly. Unfortunately, so had his confidence. At the end of the lesson he and a new swimming buddy were keen to play in the shallow, sloped end of the pool. Against my better judgement — that Mummy sixth sense we all have — I allowed him into the water unaccompanied for the first time. I gave him strict instructions not to swim past a certain point and marched up and down the side of the pool watching his every move. Technically, I was within arm's reach of him but this was presuming he could also reach out to me: a presumption I will never make again.

Following his umpteenth 'Just one more swim, Mummy', he unintentionally swam past THAT point and suddenly found himself out of his depth. Although he could touch the bottom with his tiptoes and bob his nose just above the surface, he could do nothing else. He kind of just looked at me, wide-eyed, silent, occasionally bobbing his nose above the surface. There was no panic to be seen, no arm waving or shouting, just wide-staring eyes.

It took me several seconds to realise he was in difficulty and unable to help himself. I leaned forward and called his name, encouraging him to swim to me, but he just stayed still, staring. I kneeled down and reached out to him, calling for him to reach for me, which he could have done easily. I was technically still within arm's reach but he wasn't making any effort to reach out to me. There was no one in the immediate vicinity to help him, no lifeguard, just me. It had already been about 15 seconds, so I jumped in fully clothed, pulled him towards me and put him on the side of the pool, where he sat, still wide-eyed and silent. The pool staff arrived, equally surprised, as were those parents who were sitting on the side, watching.

My child had been drowning but no one had known.

He was in shock, but otherwise fine. I was not. Guilt-ridden and soaking wet, I was just grateful I had not been distracted by my phone or his younger sister, who was strapped into her stroller.

Always watch, never presume. Drowning is silent and still, and can happen anywhere.

Sue

Respect the ocean, and stay calm if out of your depth

In my 25-year career as a lifeguard and surf educator, I have travelled the world extensively, spreading the message about surf safety. We have reduced drowning numbers exponentially in countries like India by passing on some very simple messages about how it's important to respect the ocean and know what to do if you're stuck in a rip.

One of the key things we teach young kids is the importance of learning how to float on their backs if they get out of depth. There are a lot of myths about the beach; things like collapsing sandbanks and undertows, and how rips drag you out to sea. We've used drones and GPS information to show people that 90 per cent of rips will run parallel to the beach and onto a sandbank. If you can teach your kids to stay calm and then to turn onto their back or just remain upright and calmly float, within about four minutes they will be able to stand or be near someone who is standing, where they can get help. If they are able to raise one arm they should do so. You cannot drown if your head is above water, so staying calm and floating are key.

There's a whole range of things that happen to a drowning person that people generally don't understand. You know the feeling when you're exercising and you've trained really hard and your legs feel like jelly? That's what happens to your body when you're drowning; the build-up of lactic acid is very intense. People often think that an undertow is dragging them under the water, but the reality is the body is trembling and losing energy very quickly. Again, staying calm, being educated about how to stay afloat are really important lifesaving skills.

In my business, Surf Educators International, which I run with former Iron Men Craig Riddington and Grant Kenny, we take kids as young as four years old into the water. In a controlled environment and using flotation devices such as kickboards, as well as plenty of adult supervision, we show them what to do if they are in a rip. We love it when they see how effective staying calm and floating are; it's empowering for them, and for us. It means those kids are learning how to treat the surf with knowledge and respect and not to panic if they get out of their depth.

Every backyard pool should have a flotation rescue device. Parents need to get their kids used to dragging each other around on it and reaching or throwing it out to someone who might be having trouble staying afloat. Unfortunately, often by the time paramedics arrive at the scene of a backyard pool drowning, the child is still at the bottom of the pool. With education, you can prevent this from happening.

The red and yellow flags at the beach are there for a reason. It is the safest part of the beach and this is where you need to be swimming. Unfortunately, red and yellow (red in particular) are the colours of danger, so tourists visiting Australian beaches are often confused about where they should be swimming. Similarly, in countries such as Japan, red and yellow flags signal private swimming areas, so for those visitors our red and yellow flags mean 'Stay away'! Teach your kids that the first rule of the beach is to swim between the flags. If your older kids can swim on their own, make sure you remind them to keep an eye on where they're swimming, and if they're drifting away from the flags, either to swim back or to go in to shore and walk up the beach to where the flags are.

When we rescue kids, we try to explain how they got into the position in the first place and then what to do. Sometimes the message doesn't get through because they're a bit panicked, and this is where parents come in.

Parents: the lifeguards are not a babysitting service. It's not fair on the thousands of other beachgoers to have our lifeguards relocating lost children and preventing them from getting into dangerous situations. Keep an eye on your kids. Keep young kids within arm's reach. And whatever you do, don't leave your eight- or nine-year-old in charge of your three-year-old while you go to the pub.

We do our best to look after you at the beach. We average one drowning every seven years, and that's with over 55 million people coming to the beaches we patrol over that time. It's a huge job and one that we're highly trained to do well. But as Sarah says, nothing replaces hands-on education, so make sure your kids learn about surf safety. That way you can have fun AND be safe at the beach.

Bruce 'Hoppo' Hopkins
Head Lifeguard, Bondi Beach
Deputy President,
Surf Educators International
President, Australian Professional
Lifeguard Association

EYE INJURIES

Eye injuries always make me cringe. For some reason, it's my weak spot. Eyes are just so sensitive. For a child, an eye injury can be very painful and quite scary. If your child injures her eye, you need to seek medical help.

Eye injuries can include hits or pokes to the eye, and chemicals or other substances or foreign bodies in the eye. My daughter was once playing with a glow stick she received at a party, snapped it in half and splashed the contents into her eye. (These toys are particularly dangerous, so if one makes its way to your place, quietly bin it.) Finger pokes to the eye can be the defence of choice for some feisty toddlers. One of the most common causes of eye injuries in children (be it their own or the eye of another child) is the brandishing of sticks and stick-like objects in an unsafe way.

According to the American Academy of Ophthalmology, nearly half (44.7 per cent) of all eye injuries occur in the home, with boys being three times more likely to sustain an eye injury than girls.

TYPES OF EYE INJURIES

Foreign objects

Foreign objects are anything — such as dust, glass, dirt — that doesn't belong in the eye. Foreign objects need to be flushed out with water. This is a physical challenge with most children. It is important to flush out the object with gently, as rubbing the eye can cause abrasions to the cornea (surface of the eye). Cornea abrasions can lead to infection, ulcers and possibly loss of vision.

You may have to swaddle your young child to be able to get her to cooperate. Wrap her up in a sheet and if possible enlist the help of another adult. Hold her eye open under gentle running water for five minutes then look to see if the foreign object has been flushed out. Do not force her eye open. If the object is still there or if you're unsure whether it's gone, seek medical help. If you're having difficulty flushing your child's eye with water, it's also better to seek medical help. Go to your GP or the nearest emergency department.

It is really important that you don't let your child rub her eye. If there is foreign matter or a foreign body in her eye, she can cause further damage by rubbing. To prevent this you can tape a paper or Styrofoam cup over the affected eye. Placing a pad or cloth over the eye can put pressure on the eye so they're best avoided. Besides, little hands can still rub eyes with a pad on top.

If an object has penetrated your child's eye, this is a medical emergency and you must go straight to your nearest hospital. DO NOT try to remove the embedded object. Lay your child down on her back, do not put any pressure over the eye, and use the cup method to protect it. Then call an ambulance on 000.

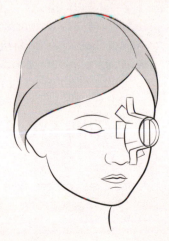

Tape a cup over the eye to prevent rubbing

Chemicals

Chemicals such as household cleaners, perfumes and beauty products can burn or irritate the eyes and need to be flushed out with running tap water. Symptoms of a chemical burn depend on what has been splashed into the eyes, but might include:

+ Stinging
+ A burning sensation
+ Redness
+ Pain
+ Swelling of the eyelids
+ An inconsolable child

If something non-toxic such as soap or shampoo gets in your child's eye/s, flush with water using the method above for 10 to 15 minutes. This feels like a very long time. If you are unsure whether the substance is toxic or an irritant, call **Poisons Information** on **13 11 26** and flush the eye with water for a minimum of 20 minutes. Make sure you wash your child's hands, as she may have spilled chemical onto them too.

When it comes to eye injuries, one of the key things is to act quickly. Medical help is usually needed so it's important to get treatment as soon as possible.

> The NSW Agency for Clinical Innovation's website is a terrific, interactive resource you can use to teach your children all about caring for their eyes and eye safety.
> Visit **www.eye playsafe.org.au**.

PREVENTING AND TREATING EYE INJURIES

Prevention

There are common-sense measures you can take to help prevent eye injuries:

+ Use appropriate safety equipment when playing sport.
+ Avoid letting your child play with projectile toys, such as darts.

+ Ensure all chemicals are kept out of reach.
+ Teach your child safety around animals, as bites to the face can often involve the eye (see **Bites & Stings**, pages 74–76).
+ Supervise children around glow sticks and other items containing the chemical dibutyl phthalate.
+ Teach your child not to throw sand or dirt at other children's faces.

Recognition

So how can you tell if your child has injured her eye? Often a child will be reluctant to let you look at her eye, or she may be constantly rubbing it. She also may show some of these signs and symptoms:

+ Complaining of pain to the eye
+ Red, watery eye
+ Pressing her eye shut
+ One eye looks different from the other
+ Sudden problems with vision
+ Cut or torn skin around the eye or eyelid
+ Light sensitivity
+ Swelling to her eyelid
+ Blood in her eye
+ Bruising on or around her eye
+ Difficulty or inability to move her eye normally
+ Squinting or excessive blinking

Response

It's easier said than done, but you need to make sure your child DOES NOT touch or rub her eye.
When administering first aid to your child, DO NOT:

+ Apply pressure to the eye.
+ Try to remove anything stuck in the eye.
+ Put any medication such as drops or ointment into the eye before getting medical help.
+ Force the eye open.

DO promptly take your child to hospital or the GP.

SUMMARY

+ Don't let your child rub her eyes, as this can make the injury worse.

+ Foreign bodies or substances splashed into the eye/s require flushing with gently running water.

+ Do not try to remove anything stuck in the eye/s; use a cup to cover the eye/s and seek urgent medical help.

'Her right eye was firmly shut and she was screaming'

When my daughter was three years old, she and I decided to spend the day doing some gardening while my wife was at work. Apart from the fact that a three-year-old puts more dirt anywhere other than in the garden, we were having a productive day. When it came time to dig holes for the plants, my daughter dug her spade in nice and deep then flicked the entire thing directly into her face. I wasn't worried about the dirt she ate, just the big dirt clods that had made it into her eyes. I managed to brush the dirt off her left eye, but her right eye was firmly shut and she was screaming. I knew that she needed to have her eye flushed out, but trying to get a kicking, screaming three-year-old to open her eye under water was impossible, and I knew not to force her eye open. If I'd had another adult with me it might have been doable, but I knew I couldn't manage it properly on my own. We went up to our local emergency department, where anaesthetic eye drops were put in and her eye was flushed with copious amounts of saline. It was lucky we did, because she had a large amount of dirt under her eyelid, which could have caused abrasions to the surface of her eye. Three years on she is still a keen gardener!

Paul

FOREIGN BODIES

Children just love to put things where they shouldn't. Toast into DVD players, credit cards into washing machines and beads into ears. If you think about every place on a child that could have something inserted into it, I can guarantee you I have seen it happen in that place. Even older children who should know better do silly things like stick Lego up their noses. Unfortunately, when kids put things up their nostrils, there is a danger that they will inhale the object or get an infection from rotting food in the nose (not pretty and smells gross, so it needs to come out). If your child has stuck something into an orifice, it is likely you will need medical help to get it out.

Prevention

Whoever said 'Never stick anything smaller than your elbow in your ears or nose' absolutely nailed it. So true, and this gem of wisdom should be imparted to all children.

Another certainty I want you to believe is this:

Kids + hole = put something in it

Some of the common objects that I've seen in children's ears and noses include food (particularly peas and corn but also popcorn, seeds and nuts), beads, pebbles and small rocks, toy parts, bits of crayon and erasers, and small batteries. I'd be mad to suggest that list has a limit, so I'll just say that pretty much anything goes for a kid who's curious enough.

The best way to prevent your child from putting things where they don't belong is to talk to her. Explain what can happen if she sticks something in her nose. Keep it simple, but make it clear: it can be painful, cause her nose to bleed or make her sick. Just saying 'Don't do it!' is like a red rag to a bull. Explain the consequences.

Keep little things that fit into noses out of reach. This doesn't help for the seven-year-old who shoves the head of a Lego figurine up his nose to impress his mates, but keeping beads out of the hands of an 18-month-old is a good idea.

Kids sometimes do things that simply defy all common sense. Like the three-year-old boy I nursed who managed to stretch his foreskin over part of a Matchbox car. Needless to say, he had to have an operation to remove it. I'm not sure who was more scarred — him or his dad!

Recognition

Children can be very sneaky when it comes to introducing foreign objects into their bodies. They know they shouldn't have put that pebble in their ear or that eraser up their nose, so the object may live up there for a while until you notice a rancid smell and discharge coming from the nose or ear. At some point, you'll hear about the pain, particularly if it involves an ear.

Small button batteries will be very painful, as they start to burn quickly. This is a medical emergency and you need to seek help urgently. Call 000 if you suspect your child has put a button battery in an orifice.

Response

As far as putting things where they shouldn't go is concerned, I have had first-hand experience through my own children. A few years ago, my younger daughter decided to put a pea up her nose. I managed to take a peek up her nostrils and, sure enough, right up the top beyond the reach of anything was a shiny green pea. She had smuggled it off her dinner plate and into the car as we were heading out. I guess she couldn't find a suitable place to store her treasure, so she decided her nose would be the spot.

Luckily, I had some tricks up my sleeve. At the hospital I have seen this method used successfully many times: block the nostril that is clear, then put your mouth completely over your child's mouth, sealing it well, and BLOW! The pressure of the air you blow in should get behind the object and hopefully cause it to fly out of your child's nostril; everything's connected in there.

I gave it a go. I sat my daughter on my lap, blocked the clear nostril and, much to her surprise, blew air into her mouth. Out of her nose came a torrent of snot and, thank goodness, a very large green pea. Mission accomplished. This technique is often referred to as the Mother's Kiss.

My daughter assured me that only one pea had gone in (verified, wide-eyed, by her older sister) but I had a thorough look just in case. We had a very serious discussion about not putting anything into any part of her body, including eyes, ears, nose, bottom and vagina. Best to cover all bases — I have seen it all in the emergency department. I am happy to say there have not been any more insertions into orifices, and I hope we keep it that way.

My daughter was not able to blow her nose independently at the time, but if your child has mastered this, you can get her to take a big breath in through her mouth, and while you are blocking the clear nostril, get her to blow her nose. This may produce enough force to pop the object out.

If this, or the Mother's Kiss, doesn't work, you will need to see a doctor. Don't try to remove the object yourself, as you can cause trauma to the inside of the nose or push the object further in. Not only that, but if your child gets upset and traumatised by your attempt, the likelihood of her then letting the doctor or nurse have a go is zero.

Generally we only have one window of opportunity to get the object out. Unless you're confident you can do it, leave it to the experts.

This is especially true for objects in ears, genitalia and eyes. (Also see **Eye Injuries**, pages 144–148.) Do not try and remove anything, just get medical help.

SUMMARY

+ If your child is combative or upset, do not try to remove it — seek medical help.

+ If the object is in your child's nose and she is calm, try one of the two blowing methods described above.

+ If neither of these blowing methods work, seek medical help.

+ Particularly seek medical help for foreign objects in ears, eyes and genitalia.

HEAD INJURIES

I wrote earlier that toddlers' big heads seem out of proportion to the rest of their little bodies. A toddler's head can be one-third the size of her body, which is quite large in comparison with an adult's. As a consequence, toddlers' heads are more prone to injury. Fortunately, however, they are also cleverly designed to withstand bumping into walls and floors. When impact occurs, large foreheads and thick skulls help protect the eyes and brain.

A head injury is defined as a knock or bump to your child's head resulting in bleeding, lumps, bumps or bruises to the head. The under-threes account for nearly half of all reported childhood head injuries.

Prevention

There are plenty of common-sense actions we can take to prevent head injuries in kids. Of course, there are accidents that we can't prevent, like that one-year-old teetering as she takes her first steps, or the five-year-old who runs into the only pole with in a 100-metre radius of where she is playing. But there are many head injuries that most definitely *can* be prevented.

The most obvious prevention method is to ensure your child ALWAYS wears a helmet while riding anything with wheels. Whether it's a bike, skateboard or other form of wheeled transport, helmet-wearing is not negotiable. Make it a rule in your house: no helmet, no wheels. End of story. But you need to go a step beyond just making your child wear her helmet: you need to ensure it fits properly as well.

Often parents or carers don't think it is necessary for a toddler to wear a helmet when on a scooter. How fast can they possibly go, right? Wrong. I have seen toddlers take big tumbles from scooters and end up with a head injury. You would be surprised at the speed a toddler can go, inevitably getting the speed wobbles, which results in a big stack. They don't even need to be going that fast to fall off and hurt their head (or another body part).

When your child is playing sport, always make sure she uses appropriate safety equipment, including a helmet. If you have stairs in your home, make sure you use a stair gate and teach your little one how to get safely up and down the stairs (on her bottom!).

Items like high chairs and prams have safety straps for a reason. Use them. I remember when my older daughter was about nine months old and she fell asleep in the car. She wasn't the best sleeper, so I was reluctant to wake her. I carefully transferred her to the pram and she started to stir when I went to click the straps on. I stopped, thinking that I would go back and click her in properly once she had settled back to sleep, but I forgot. Ten minutes later, as I was walking down the concrete driveway pushing the pram, there was an almighty thud as she sat up in the pram and fell straight out onto her head. Needless to say, I never forgot to strap her in again, asleep or awake.

Falls from change tables are another all-too-common cause of head injuries. Babies develop so quickly, so watch yours closely. You might not realise your baby can turn over by herself until she takes a tumble off the change table or bed. Always keep one hand on your baby when she is on the change table, or just keep the change mat on the floor.

Recognition

It is unusual for a toddler to become unconscious (knock herself out) from a bump to the head. If the impact is big enough to knock out your child, you need to seek urgent medical help by ringing for an ambulance on 000.

Minor head injuries tend to occur when a child hits her head and she ends up with a swelling or 'egg' at the point of impact. A minor head injury may make a young child cry for a few minutes but then she will quite happily carry on with whatever she was doing. Her behaviour will be perfectly normal. You can try to apply an ice pack to the swelling. However, many kids won't tolerate this, so a cold face washer will work just as well.

For a mild head injury, you may expect your child to show the following signs and symptoms:

+ Alert and cries immediately after the fall
+ Miserable but consolable, with a quick recovery
+ Mild, controllable headache
+ Firm egg-like lump/bump at the impact area
+ Sleeps but wakes easily
+ Minor wound or bruising
+ Normal behaviour, speech and movement

More concerning signs and symptoms you need to look out for include:

+ Loss of consciousness
+ Seizure
+ Drowsiness (outside of her normal sleep time)
+ Distressed and inconsolable
+ Headache not going away
+ A jelly-like lump on her head (boggy swelling)
+ Clear fluid or blood from nose/ears
+ Unusual behaviour
+ Two or more vomits after the injury
+ Visual disturbance

It is important that you seek urgent medical help if your child shows any of these symptoms. As I have said before, trust your instincts. If you are concerned for any reason, seek medical help.

Many parents worry about a bump on the head. How do you know what is okay and what isn't? A **boggy swelling** is a lump or swelling that is spongy or squishy to the touch. If you can feel this, it is very important to seek urgent medical help, as it can mean there is significant internal bleeding. A nurse I know has a great analogy for this: if the lump feels like an avocado that isn't quite ready to eat (firm) that is good. If the lump feels like an avocado that is overripe (only good for guacamole), that is worrying.

Response

If your child has had a head injury just prior to bedtime and she is not showing any of the above signs, it is okay to let her go to sleep. You do need to make sure you can wake her up easily, though, so check on her 10 minutes after putting her to bed. You should then check on her regularly for a couple of hours. Again, always go with your gut instincts. If you are worried, seek medical help.

The first aid for a head injury is simple:

+ Give your child a cuddle and console her, then assess the extent of the injury.
+ Keep her calm and still if it has been a significant fall.
+ Apply pressure to a bleeding wound for a minimum of 10 minutes.
+ Give pain relief, such as paracetamol, if needed.
+ Apply a cold pack to the bump if your child will tolerate it.
+ Monitor her for concerning signs.

I remember one little girl called Amelia who was prematurely ageing her parents with her love of jumping off very high things. One day she decided it might be fun to jump from the staircase to the couch and miscalculated the distance (as young children tend to do). She landed face-first on timber floorboards. She didn't lose consciousness, but her dad described her as 'stunned' for around 10 seconds before she burst into tears. She didn't appear to have any lumps, bumps or bruising but her dad said that she wasn't her normal self; she just sat on the couch very quietly, not moving, for around 30 minutes. This concerned her parents, so they brought Amelia to the emergency department. On the way she started vomiting. Amelia needed to be watched in the emergency department for a few hours, but was then sent home, as she was back to her usual self, tearing around and playing.

Amelia's parents did the right thing in taking her to hospital. Symptoms such as Amelia's signify potential for a head injury — something that most certainly needs to be assessed in hospital.

SUMMARY

If your child has any of the following symptoms after hitting her head, or you are simply concerned, you must seek urgent medical help:

+ Vomiting
+ Drowsiness outside of her normal sleep time
+ Blurred vision
+ Dizziness
+ Unusual behaviour
+ Seizure
+ Boggy swelling to the area of impact
+ Confusion
+ Persistent headache
+ Loss of consciousness

'I knew when she kept vomiting that she needed to go to the hospital'

My six-year-old daughter was playing in the driveway of our home with our neighbours one Friday afternoon. She ran into a couple of the other little kids and was knocked backwards, hitting her head on the driveway.

She initially complained of a headache, so I gave her some ibuprofen, and she settled and slept through the night.

In the morning, she was still complaining of a headache, and had a vomit. I gave her one more dose of pain relief and she seemed fine, running around, and even ate some hot chips.

That evening, while we were driving home, she vomited in the car. This was not unusual, as she often had carsickness but this time I was on alert. The next morning,

she vomited six times. I immediately took her to the emergency department, where she became drowsy. The CT scan showed that she had an extradural haematoma — blood had collected in between her skull and the protective lining that covered her brain. She was taken to the operating theatre and had a craniotomy and the blood drained away. After one night in intensive care she was moved to the ward, and made a complete recovery. Now you would not even know that the accident happened.

The important thing is to know what signs to look for. I knew when she kept vomiting that she needed to go to the hospital.

Annemarie

'No helmet, no wheels'

Working in a children's emergency department, I see plenty of injuries from a range of activities. Many of these involve kids being adventurous, pushing boundaries or simply believing they can fly. Or sometimes all of the above.

The one thing that makes me feel sick to my stomach is those kids who sustain head injuries after falls skating, riding or scootering without a helmet. These injuries can range from learning or behavioural difficulties to life-changing brain injuries — simply because they didn't wear a helmet.

For kids who come in after falling off whatever they were riding and have a pretty straightforward injury like grazes, a sprain or a broken bone — they're the lucky ones because we can fix those. For broken brains — well, that's something we can't fix.

Kids are never too old to be told to wear a lid!

Every parent's rule should be: no helmet, no wheels.

Paul
Paediatric emergency nurse

LIMB INJURIES

Broken bones, sprains and strains are common maladies of childhood. I think if you survive childhood without breaking (or at least spraining) something, you haven't played hard enough. Breaks, otherwise known as fractures, are among the most common injuries we see in the emergency department. Kids are always falling off things, particularly trampolines, monkey bars and scooters. We know we can't wrap kids up in cotton wool so, just to remind you, the key is knowing how to help if they do injure themselves.

Prevention

Children's bones are continually growing and are not yet solid like an adult's. They are 'plastic', elastic and spongy; therefore they don't often break the whole way through. Even though limb injuries are a scary thought, they are incredibly common and kids usually heal very well. Kids are more likely to injure an arm than a leg, as it is a natural reflex to put their arms out to stop a fall.

When it comes to preventing limb injuries, just like head injuries, it is important to use the right safety equipment. So make sure Santa brings the knee and elbow guards with the new skateboard, not just the helmet. A healthy diet with enough calcium and vitamin D is also essential for good bone growth and strength, as is exercise.

Recognition

So how do you know if the injury is just a sprain or if the limb is broken or dislocated? First, let's talk about the differences.

A **break or fracture** is a complete or incomplete break in a bone as a result of excessive force. These forces can be from pulling, twisting, squeezing or hitting. Breaks occur when these forces exceed the strength of the bone.

A **sprain** occurs when ligaments (strong, stretchy bands that hold bones together) are overstretched or torn, as in an ankle sprain.

A **strain** occurs when a muscle has been overstretched or torn, usually from physical movement. These are particularly common complaints after playing sport.

A **dislocation** may occur when the ligaments that hold together the ends of two bones are put under extreme force and separate. A common dislocation in children is a pulled elbow — see 'Pulled elbows' on page 162).

Babies and toddlers have stronger ligaments than bones so are more likely to break a bone than suffer a sprain or dislocation. But unless you have X-ray eyes, you won't know what type of injury it is. Sometimes a fracture can be very obvious (when the arm is shaped like a banana), and sometimes kids will still be using an arm that is fractured (and Mum will feel very guilty because it took a week to get to the doctor).

Common types of fractures in children

The most common type of fracture in kids is an incomplete fracture, meaning that the break doesn't go all the way through the bone.

Common minor fractures in kids are:

+ **Greensticks** — the bone bends and 'frays', similar to when you bend a green stick (a small branch freshly cut from a tree) and it doesn't snap.
+ **Buckles** — one side of the bone bends, resulting in a little buckle.

More serious fractures include:

+ **Open/compound fractures** — the bone breaks through the skin.
+ **Displaced fractures** — the bone breaks completely and is no longer aligned.

Both these types of fractures often need surgical intervention.

Pulled elbows

Pulled elbows are a very common injury in toddlers and children under the age of five years. A pulled elbow happens when a child is lifted up suddenly and sharply by her arm, or her arm is twisted behind her. The escaping toddler springs to mind. As she makes her getaway across a road, a parent grabs her by the arm to pull her back, and voilà! — pulled elbow. The ligament holding the arm and elbow is overstretched and the bone slips out of place.

If your child has a pulled elbow, she may be holding the arm limply down her side and be distressed only if you try to move her arm. She may complain of pain in her wrist or elbow. This requires a trip to the doctor or emergency department for assessment and a quick procedure to relocate the bone. No X-rays or follow-up are usually needed.

There are some common signs and symptoms that you need to look out for that may indicate a genuine injury to the limb. Remember, you don't have x-ray eyes so you need to look out for these signs. At the site of the injury you may see:

+ Swelling
+ Deformity
+ Bruising
+ An open fracture

Your child may feel or show:

+ Pain
+ Reluctance to move or use the limb
+ Distress when the limb is touched

The important next steps are to apply first aid and seek medical help.

Response

The principles of first aid for limb injuries are simple:

+ Immobilise and elevate the limb.
+ Apply a cold pack.
+ Give pain relief (such as paracetamol or ibuprofen).
+ Seek medical help.

If the bone is sticking out of the skin or there is a large deformity (the limb is bent), try not to move your child. Broken bones moving about on each other feel excruciatingly painful. If your child is in danger, for instance in the middle of a busy road, you may need to carefully move her to a safe place first. Otherwise, make her as comfortable as possible where she is. Call an ambulance on 000. When the paramedics arrive, they will give your child pain medication, then splint the limb, then move her. This is particularly important if her fingers or toes are cold or turning pale or blue, or your child is complaining of numbness or pins and needles. This can mean the blood supply or nerves have been damaged and it is a medical emergency.

Children can be quite stoic, so if you are concerned, apply first aid and get medical attention.

If it is not a major limb injury, you will need to apply first aid then take your child to the GP or emergency department to be reviewed.

How to immobilise a limb in a child

This can be very tricky with a child, particularly a toddler. I think slings can often be a waste of time. Children, especially toddlers, tend to let their arms dangle out or just be non-compliant. In my opinion, the best way to immobilise a child's arm is to use the clothing they are wearing. A T-shirt, singlet, dress or jumper will do the job. Lift the bottom up and over her sore arm and secure it with a knot in the back. The knot will ensure the top of her arm is tight and secure so she can't let the arm droop down. You can then apply an ice pack over the top and give some paracetamol or ibuprofen.

Little legs can be immobilised using a pillow or clothing, or anything similar you have around you. Use a bandage, scarf or piece of clothing and secure above and below the injured body part, taking care not to tie knots over the broken area.

Cold packs and elevation are very important in suspected broken bones, as they not only reduce the swelling but help with the pain too. Always give your child an analgesia, such as paracetamol or ibuprofen. Don't worry about 'masking' the symptoms; the priority is to give pain relief. Just make sure you tell the paramedic, nurse or doctor what you gave and when.

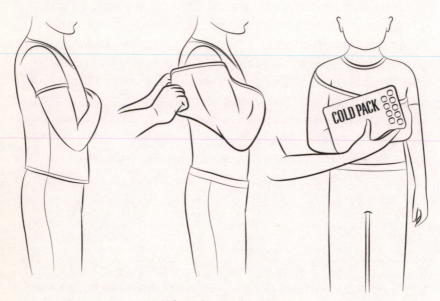

Using a jumper as a sling

Although most broken bones are quite straightforward and just need an X-ray, cast and follow-up with the doctor, bones that are badly displaced need to be repositioned. The most common way to do this with children is under a general anaesthetic. It is therefore very important not to give your child anything to eat or drink after she injures herself, just in case she needs an operation to put her bones back together in the right place.

SUMMARY

For **severe limb injuries**:

+ If the fingers or toes of the affected limb are pale, blue or cold in comparison with the other limb, or your child is complaining of numbness or pins and needles, or if there is a large deformity (the limb is bent), or the bones have come through the skin, this is a medical emergency so call an ambulance on 000.

+ Don't attempt to move your child or the limb (unless she is in danger) — just make her as comfortable as possible.

+ Don't give your child anything to eat or drink.

For **minor/moderate limb injuries**:

+ Immobilise the limb.

+ Elevate.

+ Apply a cold pack.

+ Give pain relief and seek medical help.

Trampoline injury

It was my dad's 40th birthday, and my sister and I were at home with our babysitter, Brooke. We were jumping on the trampoline and I was bouncing really high, but when I came down I fell and landed on my ankle in a weird position. She carried me up to the couch and elevated my leg. She put an ice pack on it and it hurt like mad. She gave me some medicine to make me feel better. Then Mum and Dad came home. My dad thought it was just a sprain, but then in the middle of the night when I woke up and wanted to go to the toilet, I put my foot on the ground and I screamed in pain.

The next morning both my parents took me to the children's hospital and I had an X-ray. The doctor said my ankle was broken so they put on a cast. Then a few days later when the swelling went down I got another cast. I got to choose the colour so I picked my favourite: purple.

Eva, age eight

Rough play

My two little boys, Beau, five, and Josh, three, are very active. There is a lot of rough-and-tumble in our house, and if they aren't fighting for real, they are play-fighting. We are constantly hearing either screams of laughter or screams of tears. Most of the time, the screams die off after a couple of minutes and they go back to playing normally, at least for a little while.

A few weeks ago, though, Josh ran inside screaming after Beau had pushed him to the ground. The tears were taking a little longer than usual to dry up, so we had him rest on the couch. He was complaining of pain in his shoulder and he was hesitant to lift his arm. We decided a trip to the Emergency department was the best option.

After a dose of pain relief he began to perk up, and you wouldn't have thought there was anything wrong with him. However, the X-rays revealed that he had a broken collarbone and he was immediately put into a sling.

One week later, just as he was starting to heal, he slipped over in the shower. I remember hearing that same painful cry. An immediate trip back to the emergency department and another X-ray showed that the fall had made the break worse.

It frightened me how easily his bone had broken, yet it amazed me how quickly it started to heal, and soon he was back into more rough-and-tumble with his big brother!

Rachel

'Rosie was in a lot of pain ... we both kept calm for her sake'

It was the first day of our family holiday and our 18-month-old daughter Rosie's first time on a plane. After we had landed and had breakfast, we went straight to the park. Rosie was having a great time, toddling about and playing, so I sat down to relax and enjoy watching my husband and daughter having a very happy family play. The next thing I knew I was hearing THAT cry. It was my baby's cry, but a slightly different, more painful one. I looked up to find my husband running back to me, carrying a very distressed little girl. Rosie was absolutely inconsolable. She was screaming and tensing her whole body up with even the slightest bit of movement.

My husband explained to me, in a very panicky state, that when he had gone down the slide with her, her legs had become caught underneath him. By the end of the slide, his body weight had been entirely on top of them. He was terrified he had 'snapped' her little legs. I knew that regardless of what had happened, Rosie was in a lot of pain. I happened to have some paracetamol in my bag, so after a quick dose we decided to get to the hospital — this was going to take more than a GP visit. After asking a local where the nearest hospital was, we managed to get Rosie into the car.

The trip was agonising and emotional, as she remained very distressed. On arrival, the nurse could see how much pain Rosie was in and quickly gave her some more pain relief. The next couple of hours were very tough, with X-rays, examinations and lots and lots of tears, but we both kept calm for her sake. I was, and still am, especially proud of my husband for keeping his cool in the tricky situation and managing the devastation and guilt of feeling like he had hurt his beloved little girl. Of course, it was just an accident that could have happened to anyone at any time, and no one was to blame. Rosie had a common toddler, or spiral, fracture on one leg and had two types of casts on for the next six weeks.

It was heartbreaking to see my baby in so much pain but staying calm and getting her help were the best things to do.

Emily

Know your child, and know the story behind the injury

Sometimes it's tricky to know whether your child has an injury that will heal by itself, or she needs medical attention. If there is an obvious bone break and your child is clearly distressed, then yes, you should go to your nearest emergency department. However, if your child is complaining that something 'hurts', either persistently or sporadically, you might seek help from a physiotherapist.

If you're going to see a physiotherapist, make sure they give you a clear diagnosis and communicate what timeframes are involved with recovery. Try to let your child explain the issue and the 'story' behind the discomfort. I would say the majority of paediatric courses of treatment are over one to two sessions. Very occasionally children will need ongoing treatment, but this should be explained in the initial consultation.

As far as knowing if your child needs to get medical help, I suggest the following:

1. **Know your child.** Is she someone who can be prone to exaggerating? Or is she the stoic I've-broken-my-arm-but-I-still-want-to-finish-the-soccer-game kind of kid? This will influence how you make a decision about whether to seek a physiotherapist's opinion on a problem. If a child is stoic, you may be more inclined to seek a physio's advice than for a less stoic child. Watch your child when she is not aware you are observing her. If she has a significant problem, it will not disappear when he is no longer being watched by a parent/guardian. If Jack says his arm is very sore but attempts to play handball with the kids next door, observe from a distance. If he 'carries' his arm or refuses to hit with that hand, it's likely there is something amiss.

2. **Know the story.** If your child has been pushed over in the playground and says her knee is sore, it might be best to give it a day or two to see if it settles down. If she has fallen off the monkey bars and lands on her arm and says it's very sore, it might be a good reason to see a GP, head to the emergency department or to ask a physiotherapist if it's worth having an X-ray.

Kids are robust and resilient. The two-week rule for adults with a suspected injury can be shortened to a one-week rule for kids. But the principle is the same: if a child is complaining of an issue for more than a week, it might not go away by itself. Best to seek medical advice. If a child is waking in pain, especially over consecutive nights, it's an indicator that professional help is needed. Often issues will resolve themselves within a week.

Don't be fearful of scans and X-rays. The amount of radiation in a plain X-ray on a limb is negligible. There is a similar amount on a long-haul flight!

It's best not to dismiss what your child tells you. Listen carefully to the story, determine whether it's possible there is a problem that needs attention and then communicate to the child what the plan is. A possible response to a non-urgent injury might be: 'Jack, I can see that you are upset about that sore knee after James pushed you over. How about we leave it to heal for a couple of days? I think it will get better by itself, but if not, we can talk to a physiotherapist about how to get you running fast again.'

Ben Hutton
Physiotherapist and partner at the McConnell Physiotherapy Group, Mosman, Sydney

POISONING

Have you noticed how pretty cleaning products and other chemicals look? All the colours of the rainbow. The same with medications — lots of bright colours and nice smells. Have you smelled a bottle of paracetamol lately? Must be delicious!

How could these *not* be attractive to a toddler? I remember a set of four-year-old twins who drank a decent quantity of surface cleaner. When asked why they did it, the reply was that the bottle of bright-pink cleaner looked and smelled just like the pink lemonade they'd tasted at their sister's birthday party the week before. Logical, but not good for the health.

According to the World Health Organization, poisoning is one of the leading causes of hospitalisation in children worldwide. A recent Australian Institute of Health and Welfare report showed that the rates of hospitalisation due to poisoning peak at the age of two years. It found that the most common cause of poisoning is from medications, and that the most common place where poisonings occur is in the home. The under-ones are most likely to be poisoned by plants or household products.

Prevention

Prevention is always better than cure when it comes to poisoning. (Am I starting to sound like a broken record about the prevention/cure thing?)

So how do you prevent your child from ingesting or being exposed to a harmful substance? First, know what is dangerous to children. Let's think about the things around the house that are a poisoning risk. Some are obvious, others are not.

Cleaning products and household chemicals

From surface cleaners to pool chlorine, *everything* containing chemicals needs to be locked away or kept out of reach of children. Never decant chemicals into other containers that are not clearly labelled.

One of the most dangerous things in your kitchen is the dishwasher powder (or tablets). It is often left out on the bench, or kept under the kitchen sink where little hands can easily get to it. And the tablets look like super-tasty lollies, especially the ones with little coloured balls in the centre. If your child puts one of these in her mouth, it will burn. I once looked after a little girl who swallowed part of a dishwasher tablet. It scarred her oesophagus so badly she needed multiple operations to dilate it as she grew. Please keep them out of reach. If you are reading this now and realise yours are under the kitchen sink, put the book down and move them out of reach immediately!

Eucalyptus oil is a brilliant cleaner, great for washing the floors and especially for getting sticky labels off jars. It's also the oil of choice in humidifiers when kids have a cold. But keep it out of reach, as it's a poison. It's fine in tiny quantities, like in toothpaste or medicated ointments (when used according to manufacturers' instructions), but if a child swallows eucalyptus oil, urgent emergency care is needed.

Alcohol

Alcohol is *toxic* for children. My sister-in-law got into the brandy when she was four years old. Her parents found her swinging like a monkey off a scaffold in a part of their house that was being renovated at the time. Apparently, it took some effort to get her down, at which point she proceeded to vomit and possibly pass out (depends on who is telling the story). She was very lucky that nothing too major happened. Unlike gin and tonic, alcohol and children do not mix.

Medicine

Tablets look like lollies to children. They can't differentiate between Smarties and the blood-pressure tablets that Great Aunt Mabel keeps beside her bed because she needs to take them first thing each morning.

We know to keep medicine out of reach of kids, but what about something like paracetamol? I've lost count of the number of times I've visited friends' houses, only to see a bottle of paracetamol sitting on the kitchen bench, or even in the toddler's room on the chest of drawers where the clever little thing can climb up to reach it. The reaction is usually 'But it's just paracetamol, it's sold in the supermarket! How much harm could it actually do?'

Well, it can do a lot of harm. A child who is overdosed on paracetamol can get very, *very* sick, as it causes significant liver damage. Paracetamol is a very safe drug for children and adults when used according to the directions on the bottle. It is very dangerous when overdosed.

Ladies, think about your handbag. Do you have painkillers or maybe hay-fever tablets in there? A crawling child or toddler will often make a beeline for a handbag on the ground and those clever little fingers can definitely undo zips. Keep your bag out of reach.

Herbal or mineral supplements and vitamins are medicines too. They also need to be kept out of reach. Remember, a child's body is much smaller than ours. One extra tablet in an adult might be okay, but one tablet in a child may be a significant overdose.

Plants

In Australia, not only do we have some of the most venomous creatures on the planet, but we have plenty of toxic plants too. Some of the more common are oleander (*Nerium oleander*), deadly nightshade (*Atropa belladonna*) and angel trumpets (*Brugmansia* spp. or *Datura* spp.). Other common ones you don't want your little one munching on are daffodil and other *Narcissus* varieties, lily of the valley, and even the good old agapanthus. This list is by no means complete — you could write an entire book on this subject. The message is simple, though: unless you know it is food, don't eat it.

A grandfather in one of my classes could attest to the dangers of the oleander tree. He jovially told the story of when he was a 'young whippersnapper' on the farm and needed something to stir his billy tea with, so he snapped off a twig from the oleander and used that. For two days, he had severe abdominal pain and vomiting. Every part of the oleander is toxic, from the flowers to the sap. If you have an oleander plant in your garden, no need to chop it down, just make sure the kids don't eat it (and don't burn it either — even the fumes are toxic). I remember when I was very young my grandmother told me not to pick the flowers from her oleander tree because they would make me sick. From that point I gave them a wide berth.

Angel trumpets are also very common and are rather beautiful. I have seen children who pick the lovely bell-shaped flowers and pretend to use them as trumpets, but get a little too enthusiastic and have a chew on the flower too. Once again, not a good idea. Ingestion of the flower can cause abdominal pain, confusion, hallucination, intense thirst and seizures.

Recognition

When it comes to poisoning, kids can be quite sneaky. Often they know they shouldn't be drinking that particular substance, and may try to hide it from you. The first thing you might see is your little treasure with an open bottle of paracetamol and some sticky lips.

Poisoning doesn't just happen by swallowing a substance; it can be through contact (with the skin or eye/s) or inhalation (a gas or powder, for example).

Always be prepared for DRSABCD (see **CPR**, pages 30–47). Even if your child isn't showing any signs of poisoning or you aren't even sure whether she actually managed to get some of the substance down, you need to implement first aid IMMEDIATELY.

Poisons Information Line — 13 11 26

Response

If your child is unresponsive, you must immediately follow DRSABCD, ensuring you are safe and aren't going to be poisoned too.

Otherwise, the very first thing you are going to do is remove the substance from your child. A friend of mine told me about the time her 22-month-old son drank from a bottle of ibuprofen. The lid wasn't on — she had just given him a dose because he had an ear infection. She turned around to see him sitting on the kitchen bench with the syrup dripping down his chin and a cheeky grin on his face. In her panic, she immediately called the Poisons Information Line. She remembered to take the bottle from him but didn't wipe up the big puddle that he'd managed to spill. While she was relaying the event to the Poisons Information Line operator, he started to lap up the spilled syrup that was on the bench, like a dog drinking! So, before calling the Poisons Information Line, make sure to wipe up the spilled substance or remove your child from the area. Again, when it comes to chemicals, make sure you are safe too.

Take the container with you, and call the **Poisons Information Line** on **13 11 26. Put this book down and save the number into your phone now.** The person on the other end will want to know the age of your child (weight too if you know it), what poison they have been exposed to, how much there was and when the poisoning took place.

SUMMARY

If your child has INHALED poison:

+ Keep yourself safe and get you and your child into the fresh air.
+ Call the Poisons Information Line on 13 11 26.

If your child has SWALLOWED poison:

+ Remove the rest of the poison, or remove your child from the area.
+ Do not make her vomit — this can cause more damage on the way up again.
+ Call Poisons Information Line on 13 11 26 and, if possible, have the container in your hand.

If there is poison in the EYE/S or on the SKIN:

+ Remove clothing that may be contaminated with the poison, and keep yourself safe while doing so.
+ Flush the skin or eye/s with copious amounts of cool water (see **Eye Injuries**, pages 144–148).
+ Call the Poisons Information Line on 13 11 26.

Remember, if your child is unresponsive or very unwell, follow DRSABCD and call an ambulance on 000.

Keep medication safely out of reach

My 11-month-old son was seriously into exploring cupboards, and on one particular morning had discovered a bottle of prescription-strength anti-inflammatory tablets that belonged to my husband, who had recently had a knee operation.

When I found my son with the pink-coloured tablets strewn around him on the floor, I couldn't believe he had managed to open the container (yes, at 11 months old!).

I instantly went into alert mode and the first thing I did was check his mouth. He had squirrelled five tablets away in his cheeks and lips. I had no idea how many he had actually swallowed.

I called my paediatric nurse friend, who advised me to stay calm and immediately call the Poisons Information Line (and not to murder my husband, who had left the medication on a low shelf, easily accessible to the baby).

The Poisons Information Line staff were not alarmed. They reassured me and asked me how long ago it had happened, and whether he had vomited. They advised me to monitor him and to seek medical help if he started vomiting or had a significant change in behaviour. Fortunately, was absolutely fine.

Any medication in our house is now always kept very high up — completely out of reach of my curious children!

Tanya

FIRST AID QUICK REFERENCE SECTION

REMEMBER: STAY CALM. TRUST YOUR INSTINCTS. ALWAYS SEEK MEDICAL HELP IF YOU ARE CONCERNED ABOUT YOUR CHILD.

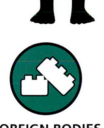
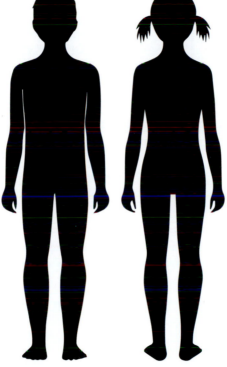
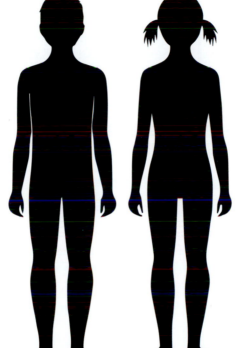

ANAPHYLAXIS

ASTHMA

BASIC LIFE SUPPORT

BITES & STINGS

SEIZURES

BLEEDING

POISONING

BURNS

LIMB INJURY

CHOKING

HEAD INJURIES

FOREIGN BODIES

EYE INJURIES

DENTAL INJURIES

RED FLAGS featured throughout this section indicate that urgent medical help is needed. Call an ambulance on 000. Follow DRSABCD and apply first aid. Do not give your child anything to eat or drink.

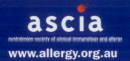

ascia
australasian society of clinical immunology and allergy

www.allergy.org.au

ACTION PLAN FOR
Anaphylaxis

For EpiPen® adrenaline (epinephrine) autoinjectors

How to give EpiPen®

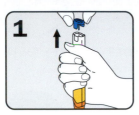

1

Form fist around EpiPen® and
PULL OFF BLUE SAFETY RELEASE

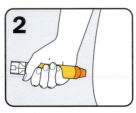

2

Hold leg still and PLACE ORANGE
END against outer mid-thigh
(with or without clothing)

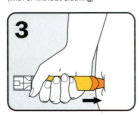

3

PUSH DOWN HARD until a click is
heard or felt and hold in place for
3 seconds

REMOVE EpiPen®

All EpiPen®s should be held in place
for 3 seconds regardless of instructions
on device label

SIGNS OF MILD TO MODERATE ALLERGIC REACTION

- Swelling of lips, face, eyes
- Hives or welts
- Tingling mouth
- Abdominal pain, vomiting (these are signs of anaphylaxis for insect allergy)

ACTION FOR MILD TO MODERATE ALLERGIC REACTION

- For insect allergy - flick out sting if visible
- For tick allergy - freeze dry tick and allow to drop off
- Stay with person and call for help
- Locate EpiPen® or EpiPen® Jr adrenaline autoinjector
- Phone family/emergency contact

Mild to moderate allergic reactions (such as hives or swelling) may not always occur before anaphylaxis

WATCH FOR ANY ONE OF THE FOLLOWING SIGNS OF ANAPHYLAXIS (SEVERE ALLERGIC REACTION)

- **Difficult/noisy breathing**
- **Swelling of tongue**
- **Swelling/tightness in throat**
- **Wheeze or persistent cough**
- **Difficulty talking and/or hoarse voice**
- **Persistent dizziness or collapse**
- **Pale and floppy (young children)**

ACTION FOR ANAPHYLAXIS

1 Lay person flat - do NOT allow them to stand or walk
  - If unconscious, place in recovery position
  - If breathing is difficult allow them to sit

2 Give EpiPen® or EpiPen® Jr adrenaline autoinjector
3 Phone ambulance - 000 (AU) or 111 (NZ)
4 Phone family/emergency contact
5 Further adrenaline doses may be given if no response after 5 minutes
6 Transfer person to hospital for at least 4 hours of observation

If in doubt give adrenaline autoinjector

Commence CPR at any time if person is unresponsive and not breathing normally

EpiPen® is prescribed for children over 20kg and adults. EpiPen®Jr is prescribed for children 10-20kg

ALWAYS give adrenaline autoinjector FIRST, and then asthma reliever puffer if someone with known asthma and allergy to food, insects or medication has SUDDEN BREATHING DIFFICULTY (including wheeze, persistent cough or hoarse voice) even if there are no skin symptoms

Kids' First Aid for Asthma

NationalAsthma
CouncilAustralia
leading the attack against asthma

1 Sit the child upright.
Stay calm and reassure the child.
Don't leave the child alone.

2 Give 4 separate puffs of a reliever inhaler – blue/grey puffer (e.g. Ventolin, Asmol or Airomir)

Use a spacer, if available.
Give one puff at a time with 4–6 breaths after each puff.

Use the child's own reliever inhaler if available.
If not, use first aid kit reliever inhaler or borrow one.

OR

Give 2 separate doses of a Bricanyl inhaler
If a puffer is not available, you can use Bricanyl for **children aged 6 years and over**, even if the child does not normally use this.

3 Wait 4 minutes.
If the child still cannot breathe normally, **give 4 more puffs.**
Give one puff at a time (Use a spacer, if available).

Wait 4 minutes.
If the child still cannot breathe normally, **give 1 more dose.**

4 If the child still cannot breathe normally,

CALL AN AMBULANCE IMMEDIATELY (DIAL 000)

Say that a child is having an asthma attack.

Keep giving reliever.

Give 4 separate puffs every 4 minutes until the ambulance arrives.

If child still cannot breathe normally,
CALL AN AMBULANCE IMMEDIATELY (DIAL 000)
Say that a child is having an asthma attack.

Keep giving reliever
Give one dose every 4 minutes until the ambulance arrives.

HOW TO USE INHALER

WITH SPACER
Use spacer if available*

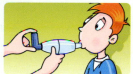

- **Assemble spacer** (attach mask if under 4)
- **Remove puffer cap and shake well**
- Insert puffer upright into spacer
- Place mouthpiece between child's teeth and seal lips around it OR place mask over child's mouth and nose forming a good seal
- **Press once firmly** on puffer to fire one puff into spacer
- **Child takes 4–6 breaths** in and out of spacer
- **Repeat** 1 puff at a time until 4 puffs taken – remember to shake the puffer before each puff
- **Replace cap**

*If spacer not available for child under 7, cup child's/helper's hands around child's nose and mouth to form a good seal. Fire puffer through hands into air pocket. Follow steps for WITH SPACER.

WITHOUT SPACER
Kids over 7 if no spacer

- **Remove cap and shake well**
- Get child to **breathe out** away from puffer
- Place mouthpiece between child's teeth and seal lips around it
- Ask child to take slow deep breath
- **Press once firmly** on puffer while child breathes in
- Get child to hold breath for at least 4 seconds, then breathe out slowly away from puffer
- **Repeat** 1 puff at a time until 4 puffs taken – remember to shake the puffer before each puff
- **Replace cap**

BRICANYL
For children 6 and over only

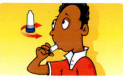

- **Unscrew cover** and remove
- **Hold inhaler upright and twist grip** around then back
- Get child to **breathe out** away from inhaler
- Place mouthpiece between child's teeth and seal lips around it
- Ask child to take a **big strong breath in**
- Ask child to breathe out slowly **away from inhaler**
- **Repeat** to take a second dose – remember to twist the grip both ways to reload before each dose
- **Replace cover**

Not Sure if it's Asthma?
CALL AMBULANCE IMMEDIATELY (DIAL 000)
If the child stays conscious and their main problem seems to be breathing, follow the asthma first aid steps. Asthma reliever medicine is unlikely to harm them even if they do not have asthma.

Severe Allergic Reactions
CALL AMBULANCE IMMEDIATELY (DIAL 000)
Follow the child's Action Plan for Anaphylaxis if available. If you know that the child has severe allergies and seems to be having a severe allergic reaction, use their adrenaline autoinjector (e.g. EpiPen, Anapen) before giving asthma reliever medicine.

For more information on asthma visit: Asthma Foundations www.asthmaaustralia.org.au   National Asthma Council Australia www.nationalasthma.org.au
If an adult is having an asthma attack, you can follow the above steps until you are able to seek medical advice.

MSC352

BASIC LIFE SUPPORT — DRSABCD

BASIC LIFE SUPPORT

D Dangers – are there any?

R Response – is your child unresponsive?

S Send for Help

A Airway – is it open?

B Breathing – is it abnormal?

C CPR
30 compressions to 2 breaths
If unwilling/unable to perform
rescue breaths continue chest
compressions

D Defibrillator – attach AED
as soon as available and
follow its prompts

INFANT

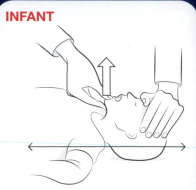

Neutral head position for infant

**Two-finger position for
infant compressions**

CHILD

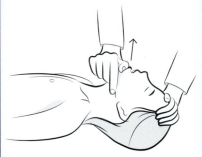

Head tilt chin lift for child

**One- or two-hand position for
child compressions**

Continue CPR until child responds or normal breathing returns

AMBULANCE 000

BITES & STINGS

FUNNEL-WEB SPIDER AND SNAKE BITES

+ If you suspect your child has been bitten by a snake or dangerous spider (see pages 85–92), call an ambulance on **000**.
+ Apply pressure bandage from bottom of bitten limb (i.e. fingers or toes) to top of limb (e.g. groin).
+ Immobilise limb.
+ For bites to the torso or neck: apply firm pressure over bite site with a cloth pad and do **not** restrict breathing.
+ Keep child completely still – do not allow her to walk around.
+ Do not wash or suck bite site.

REDBACK AND OTHER SPIDER BITES

+ Apply ice to bite area – do not apply pressure bandage.
+ Seek medical help.

BEE/WASP STINGS

+ Remove the sting promptly.
+ Wash area with soap and water.
+ Apply ice pack or cold compress.

 RED FLAGS – BEE/WASP STING

+ **ALLERGY TO BEE/WASP STINGS**
+ **DIFFICULTY BREATHING**
+ **SWELLING TO FACE, MOUTH OR TONGUE**
+ **VOMITING AND/OR ABDOMINAL PAIN**
+ **SEVERE PAIN AT STING SITE**

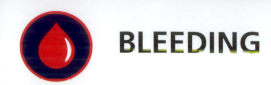

BLEEDING

WOUNDS

+ Apply firm direct pressure over the wound using clean and dry material.

+ Keep pressure on for 5 minutes.

+ If blood is spurting from the wound, apply firm direct pressure and call **000.**

+ Don't pull out anything that could be deeply embedded in a wound – stabilise the wound and seek medical help.

+ If gaping, dirty, deep or in a tricky area such as the lip, eye or ear, seek medical help.

+ Don't give your child anything to eat or drink until she is seen by a doctor.

+ If the wound is minor, clean it, apply an antiseptic of your choice if necessary and cover.

ABRASIONS (GRAZES)

+ Wash the wound with water and remove dirt.

+ Apply the antiseptic of your choice and a non-stick dressing if needed.

+ Look for signs of infection.

+ Seek medical help if you are concerned.

AMPUTATIONS

+ The priority is to apply firm direct pressure to stop or slow the bleeding.

+ Call **000**.

+ Recover the amputated part and place in damp (not wet) gauze or paper towel and seal in a plastic bag.

+ Place on an ice slurry (do not put the part directly in ice or water).

+ Amputated part to remain with the injured child.

NOSEBLEEDS

+ Keep your child calm.

+ Lean her forward.

+ Pinch her nostrils and ask her to breathe through her mouth.

+ Put a cold compress over the bridge of her nose.

+ Hold for 10 minutes.

+ DO NOT sniff, pick at or blow nose for at least 15 minutes after bleeding stops.

+ Seek medical help if the bleeding does not stop.

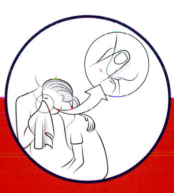

 RED FLAGS

+ **UNCONTROLLED BLEEDING**
+ **BLOOD SPURTING FROM WOUND**
+ **LARGE AND/OR DEEP WOUNDS**
+ **SEVERE PAIN**
+ **NUMBNESS/PINS AND NEEDLES TO AFFECTED BODY PART**
+ **EMBEDDED OBJECT**
+ **YOU ARE VERY CONCERNED**
+ **AMPUTATION**

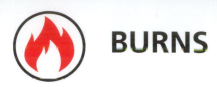

BURNS

+ For flame burns: STOP, DROP, COVER, ROLL (stop, drop to the ground, cover your face, and roll over and over).

+ Remove clothing unless it is stuck to the skin, including the nappy.

+ Cool the burn with cool, running tap water for a minimum of 20 minutes.

+ Cover the burn with cling wrap or a non-stick dressing.

+ Seek medical help.

+ You can apply first aid for up to 3 hours after the burn, and it will still be effective.

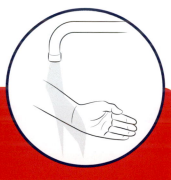

RED FLAGS

+ **BURNS TO THE FACE OR NECK**

+ **SOOT AROUND NOSE OR MOUTH – INDICATES POSSIBLE BURN INJURY TO THE AIRWAY**

+ **DIFFICULTY BREATHING**

+ **LARGE BURN AREA**

+ **SEVERE PAIN**

+ **CHEMICAL OR ELECTRICAL BURN**

+ **POSSIBILITY OF SMOKE INHALATION**

+ **WHITE, LEATHERY OR CHARRED BURN AREA**

+ **YOU ARE VERY CONCERNED**

CHOKING

IF YOUR CHILD IS UNCONSCIOUS:

+ Call an ambulance on **000**.

+ Commence basic life support (DRSABCD).

IF YOUR CHILD IS CONSCIOUS BUT IS SILENT OR UNABLE TO COUGH:

+ Give up to 5 back blows.

+ If back blows are not effective, give up to 5 chest thrusts.

+ Call an ambulance on **000** if obstruction does not clear.

+ Continue back blows/chest thrusts until airway clears/help arrives.

+ If child becomes unconscious, commence basic life support (DRSABCD).

IF YOUR CHILD IS CONSCIOUS AND HAS AN EFFECTIVE COUGH:

+ Encourage coughing.

+ Stay with child until recovery.

+ If condition deteriorates, call an ambulance on **000** and commence back blows/chest thrusts/basic life support as appropriate.

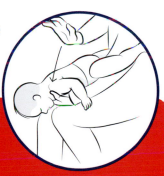

 ## RED FLAGS

+ **SILENCE OR INABILITY TO COUGH**

+ **BLUENESS IN THE FACE**

+ **EXCESSIVE DROOLING**

+ **HOARSE VOICE OR CRYING**

+ **A PERSISTENT COUGH**

+ **LABOURED OR NOISY BREATHING**

+ **IRRITABILITY OR PANIC**

DENTAL INJURIES

FOR INJURY TO OR LOSS OF A DECIDUOUS (BABY) TOOTH:

+ Pick up the tooth by the crown.

+ DO NOT touch the root.

+ Put the tooth in milk or saliva, not water.

+ DO NOT put the tooth back into the socket.

+ Go to your dentist or an emergency dental service.

FOR INJURY TO OR LOSS OF A PERMANENT TOOTH:

+ Pick up the tooth by the crown.

+ DO NOT touch the root.

+ Rinse gently in milk, saliva or saline if the root is dirty;
  DO NOT scrub or wash in water.

+ Place the tooth back into the socket if possible.

+ Get your child to bite down on a clean cloth.

+ Put the tooth in milk, saline solution or
  saliva if you cannot put it back into the socket.

+ Seek urgent dental help.

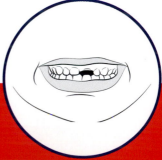

 RED FLAGS

+ **SEVERE INJURIES TO THE MOUTH OR FACE**
+ **INABILITY TO SWALLOW**
+ **DIFFICULTY BREATHING**
+ **UNCONTROLLED BLEEDING**

EYE INJURIES

+ DO NOT let your child rub her eyes.
+ Foreign bodies or substances splashed into the eye require flushing with gentle running water for 15 minutes.
+ DO NOT try to remove anything stuck in the eye.
+ DO NOT force the eye open.
+ Use a paper cup to cover the eye and seek urgent medical help.
+ Do not apply any drops or ointments before seeking medical help.

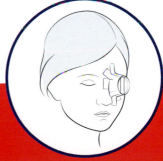

 RED FLAGS

+ **CHEMICALS OR OTHER IRRITANTS IN THE EYE**
+ **CUTS OR PUNCTURES TO THE EYE**
+ **FOREIGN BODIES IN THE EYE**

FOREIGN BODIES

+ If your child is combative or upset, DO NOT try to remove it – seek medical help.

+ If your child is calm and the object is in her nose, try the blowing method.

+ If the blowing method does not work, seek medical help.

+ Seek medical help for objects in ears, eyes and genitalia.

Foreign Body Airway Obstruction (Choking)

ASSESS

Ineffective Cough
Severe airway obstruction

Effective Cough
Mild airway obstruction

Unresponsive

Send for help
Start CPR

Responsive

Send for help

Give up to 5 back blows

If not effective give up to 5 chest thrusts

Encourage coughing

Continue to check regularly

Send for help if condition deteriorates

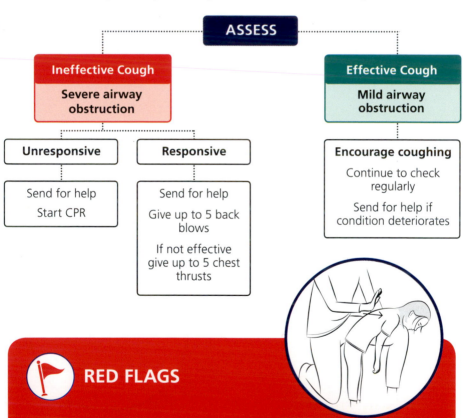

RED FLAGS

+ **DIFFICULTY BREATHING**
+ **EXCESSIVE DROOLING**
+ **INABILITY TO SWALLOW**
+ **HOARSE VOICE**

HEAD INJURIES

If your child has any of the following symptoms after hitting her head, or you are simply concerned, you must seek urgent medical help:

+ Vomiting

+ Drowsiness outside of her normal sleep time

+ Blurred vision

+ Dizziness

+ Unusual behaviour

+ Seizure

+ Boggy swelling to the area of impact

+ Confusion

+ Headache

+ Loss of consciousness

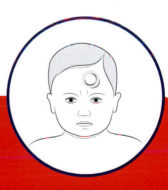

 RED FLAGS

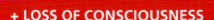

+ **LOSS OF CONSCIOUSNESS**

+ **SEIZURE (FIT)**

+ **UNCONTROLLED BLEEDING TO WOUND**

+ **DROWSINESS**

+ **INJURY CAUSED BY FALL FROM SIGNIFICANT HEIGHT OR AT HIGH SPEED**

+ **YOU ARE VERY CONCERNED**

LIMB INJURIES

SEVERE

+ If the fingers or toes of the affected limb are pale, blue or cold in comparison with the other limb, or your child is complaining of numbness or pins and needles to the injured limb, call an ambulance on **000**.

+ If there is a large deformity or the bones have pierced through the skin, this is a medical emergency. Call an ambulance on **000**.

+ Don't attempt to move your child or the limb (unless she is in danger, then do so carefully), just make her as comfortable as possible.

+ Don't give your child anything to eat or drink.

MINOR

+ Immobilise the limb.

+ Elevate.

+ Apply a cold pack.

+ Give pain relief and seek medical help.

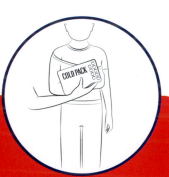

 RED FLAGS

+ **DEFORMED LIMB**
+ **OPEN FRACTURE**
  (BONES HAVE COME THROUGH THE SKIN)
+ **INJURED LIMB PALE, BLUE OR COLD IN COMPARISON**
  WITH THE OTHER LIMB
+ **PINS AND NEEDLES OR NUMBNESS**
  IN THE INJURED LIMB
+ **UNCONTROLLABLE PAIN**
+ **YOU ARE VERY CONCERNED**

POISONING

IF YOUR CHILD HAS INHALED POISON:

+ Keep yourself safe and get you and your child to fresh air.
+ Call the **Poisons Information Line** on **13 11 26**.

IF YOUR CHILD HAS SWALLOWED POISON:

+ Remove the rest of the poison, or remove your child from the area.
+ DO NOT make your child vomit — this can cause more damage as it travels back up again.
+ Call the **Poisons Information Line** on **13 11 26** and if possible have the container in your hand.

IF THERE IS POISON IN THE EYE OR ON THE SKIN:

+ Remove clothing that may be contaminated by the poison, and keep yourself safe while doing so.
+ Flush the eye or skin with copious amounts of cool running water.
+ Call the **Poisons Information Line** on **13 11 26**.

Remember, if your child is unresponsive or very unwell, follow DRSABCD and call an ambulance on **000**.

 RED FLAGS

+ **YOUR CHILD HAS DIFFICULTY BREATHING**
+ **SHE IS UNCONSCIOUS**
+ **SHE IS DROWSY**
+ **THE POISONS INFORMATION LINE TELLS YOU TO CALL FOR AN AMBULANCE**

SEIZURES

+ Keep calm.

+ Stay with your child.

+ Move your child away from danger.

+ Roll your child into the recovery position (on her side) if possible and place something soft under her head.

+ DO NOT put anything into your child's mouth.

+ Seek medical help or call an ambulance on **000**.

+ If possible, note the length of time of the seizure.

+ Commence basic life support (DRSABCD) if your child continues to be unresponsive after the seizure stops.

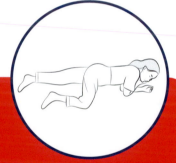

RED FLAGS

+ **FIRST SEIZURE**

+ **SEIZURE NOT STOPPING AFTER 5 MINUTES**

+ **SEIZURE DIFFERENT FROM USUAL***

+ **YOUR CHILD HAS INJURED HERSELF DURING THE SEIZURE**

+ **YOUR CHILD HAS VOMITED DURING THE SEIZURE**

+ **YOUR CHILD HAS BREATHING DIFFICULTIES AFTER THE SEIZURE STOPS**

+ **YOUR CHILD REMAINS VERY SLEEPY FOR MORE THAN 5 MINUTES AFTER THE SEIZURE STOPS**

+ **YOU ARE VERY CONCERNED**

*If your child has a diagnosed seizure disorder, remember to follow her personal action plan.

SEIZURES

A seizure, often called a fit or convulsion, is defined as a disruption in the normal pattern of the electrical impulses in the brain, caused by a surge in the electrical activity. Seizures can be subtle or very obvious. Someone having a seizure can experience jerking movements, or changes in awareness, behaviour or sensation.

There are many different reasons why a child may have a seizure. Often seizures are a symptom of another problem such as a head injury, meningitis or a fast rise in body temperature. Other times they can be part of a disease such as epilepsy.

Recognition

There are many different types of seizure and they can present in various ways. Sometimes they involve shaking of the arms and legs, other times the child may be quite stiff. However, in most cases, the child is unresponsive throughout the episode.

If your child is diagnosed with a seizure disorder, your specialist will give you an action and treatment plan specifically for your child. If your child has a seizure for the first time, you must apply first aid and call an ambulance on 000.

One very common type of seizure in children is a **febrile convulsion**, also known as a **fever seizure**. About three per cent of children aged between six months and six years will have a convulsion when there is a rapid rise in body temperature (above 38 degrees Celsius), usually associated with a fever (see **Fever**, pages 198–205). It's believed the rapid change in temperature disrupts the activity of the brain, causing the seizure. A febrile convulsion usually lasts for less than five minutes and stops without any intervention.

While febrile convulsions are benign, meaning they won't do any damage to your child's brain, it can be very scary to see your child have a seizure, particularly for the first time. Many children only ever have a single seizure. Some children will have several seizures, usually during illnesses that create a fever. There is no increased risk of epilepsy in children who have febrile convulsions.

Response

In the past, it was believed that a person having a seizure might swallow their tongue, so first aid involved sticking something such as a ruler in the mouth for them to bite down on.

DO NOT put anything into your child's mouth if she is having a seizure.

Your child cannot swallow her tongue. Some parents are concerned that their child might bite her tongue, but if this does happen the bite is usually quite minor. If *you* try to stick your fingers in your child's mouth while she is having a seizure you will probably end up needing stitches to fix the bites!

If your child has a seizure, you need to:

+ Stay with her.
+ Move her away from danger.
+ Roll her into the recovery position if possible (immediately if she has vomit, food or fluid in her mouth) and place something soft under her head.
+ NOT put anything into your child's mouth.
+ Seek medical help or call 000 for an ambulance.
+ If possible, write down the length of time of the seizure.

Your baby or child may be quite grumpy and sleepy after a seizure, and this is normal. She needs time to rest. If your child has a seizure disorder and it is taking longer than usual for her to wake up, or the seizure was different from usual, follow your action plan and seek medical help. If your child remains unresponsive when the seizure stops, commence DRSABCD immediately (see **CPR**, pages 30–47).

One of the most important things to remember if your child is having a seizure is to remain calm. It will help the doctors and nurses so much later if you can give them an accurate description of what your child was doing during the seizure and how long it lasted. Remember, in an emergency, one minute will seem like 10. Timing the seizure is very helpful, and if there is another person with you, video-recording the seizure is very helpful too.

SUMMARY

+ Keep calm.
+ Stay with your child.
+ Apply first aid. (See procedure descibed on previous page.)
+ If possible, note the length of the seizure.
+ Follow DRSABCD if your child continues to be unresponsive after the seizure stops.

A febrile seizure

I still remember Timothy's first febrile seizure. He was 10 months old and already a bit snuffly with a cold. He woke in the middle of the night and when I checked on him, he just seemed so unwell. Trusting my maternal instincts, I decided it would be best to take him to the emergency department for a check-up.

I had just walked into the building when I suddenly felt his body stiffen and arch back. I couldn't tell if he was breathing. His eyes had rolled into the back of his head and his face was twitching. I felt very shocked and scared, and even though there were nurses just a few feet away, I froze. Luckily, they acted quickly and grabbed him from my arms, rushing him off to be treated.

It took me quite a few days and quite a few buckets of tears to process the situation. Timothy is now three and a half and still gives me the occasional fright. However, I am now armed with first-aid knowledge and feel much more confident in handling his seizures. I know how to keep myself calm in the situation and spring into action. I can time the seizure and make sure he is safe. I feel much more in control now that I know what to do, but still give myself the chance to cry it out when everything is done.

Raien

PART 4

COMMON ILLNESSES IN BABIES & CHILDREN

THE GENERALLY UNWELL CHILD

Your baby is unable to tell you when something hurts, or when she feels sick. The exception to this is of course a piercing scream or distressed cry immediately after an obvious accident or injury. When nothing is *obvious*, though, it can be tricky to work out what is going on. But there are some signs and symptoms that you can look for to tell if something is wrong.

The first thing you need to understand is that *no one knows a child the way her parents do*. Parents know what is normal for their child. They know their child's rhythms and moods and when something is just 'not right'. This is so important. Even hospital staff or your doctor don't know your child like you do. What they see as unusual might be completely normal for your child, or something that might be okay in another child is a big red flag for yours. This is your litmus test.

Sometimes sick babies and kids don't have a clear set of symptoms; sometimes they do. Take a cold, for example. Your child might have a runny nose, be coughing a lot and have a mild fever. Other times, it might not be obvious that anything is wrong, but you just know that things aren't normal. In the case of a more serious infection, it's possible that your child might not have any specific symptoms until she is very, very unwell. Take meningococcal disease, for example. The rash that doesn't go away when you press on it, although very concerning, is not usually the first symptom you will see. Usually you will see other signs and symptoms first.

There are five red flags that can indicate your child is unwell and needs medical help, *sometimes urgently*. As parents and carers, if you can recognise these red flags early and seek appropriate medical help, it may just save a life.

Recognition

What are these red flags? Particularly in babies, this is what you may see:

1. Paleness
A sick child will usually have a colour change to their skin. No matter what colour skin she has, she can become quite pale in comparison with her normal colour. If your child's skin becomes grey, blue or mottled, this is even more worrying.

2. Floppiness
A very sick child may be floppy in your arms, almost like a rag doll. This is a very concerning sign.

3. Lethargy
A very sick child may be drowsy. She may be sleeping more than usual, or difficult to rouse from sleep. She may have a weak cry, or not be crying at all. She may also be unsettled and unable to be consoled.

4. Reduced feeding
A child who is taking less than half of her usual feeds in 24 hours may be very sick. She may be refusing to feed, or she may be not waking for feeds.

5. Reduced urine output
If your child has fewer than half her normal number of wet nappies over 24 hours, this is concerning.

Response

A child showing any of these signs and symptoms needs urgent medical review. A few years ago, both my daughters caught a bacterial throat infection. My youngest was alert, flushed in the cheeks, sitting up, watching TV and asking for icy poles, and had had a heavy, wet nappy that morning. My oldest daughter was pale, could not lift her head off the pillow, was falling asleep every few minutes, was refusing to drink and had not done a wee since the night before. I took her to the hospital — she was very sick. My youngest, on the other hand, needed only to go to the GP.

So, how do you respond? You need to look at your child as a whole and trust your instincts. If your child is showing any of the red flags on the previous page, you need urgent medical help. If she is unresponsive, drowsy, floppy, blue, grey, mottled, or having difficulty breathing, you need to call for an ambulance on 000 immediately.

Trust your instincts. You know your child best. If you feel like there is something wrong, you are likely to be right. Seek medical help.

'Brooke had broken out in a blue/purple rash, usually associated with meningitis'

We remember the night well. Our daughter, Brooke, was four months old. It was a Wednesday (State of Origin night) and friends had come over to our place for dinner. Brooke was an incredibly easy, settled baby and, as usual, had gone to bed without a fuss. But as our friends were leaving, she woke up and wouldn't go back to sleep unless she was being held upright against one of us. We spent the night tag-teaming and any time we tried to lie her down in her cot, she would immediately start crying and sometimes even screaming. The only way to comfort her was to cuddle her in an upright position. It was completely out of character, and by 5 a.m., we were both exhausted and knew something just wasn't right.

Luckily, we lived only five minutes' drive from our nearest hospital, and at triage we were quickly ushered through to a doctor. There were no obvious signs other than the fact Brooke did not want to be laid down. Because of this, the diagnosis was difficult, so the doctor ordered blood tests to see if this would show anything definitive.

We remember feeling not so worried, but soon after the blood tests, the doctor came to tell us that they thought Brooke had meningitis and they would have to immediately do a lumbar puncture, which would confirm whether Brooke had the disease and whether it was a viral or bacterial strain. While having the initial blood tests, Brooke had broken out in a blue/purple rash, usually associated with meningitis. She was immediately put onto round-the-clock treatment, as the results of the lumbar puncture wouldn't be known for at least three days — so the treatment had to cover all possible bases.

Fourteen days later, Brooke was released from hospital. Over the next year we had routine checks to make sure her hearing had not been affected. Fortunately, due to the quick and thorough response of the hospital, Brooke had no lasting damage to her health.

Paul & Anneka

DIARRHOEA, VOMITING & DEHYDRATION

Let's face it, at some stage in your parenting life you are going to be confronted with a vomiting, pooing mess when your child gets gastroenteritis (gastro). If you're really unlucky, the whole family ends up succumbing to the illness. There is nothing quite like caring for a spewing, squirting child (or more) whilst you are feeling like death warmed up yourself. Not pretty. But there are some things you can do to try to prevent the spread.

Gastroenteritis is an infection resulting in inflammation of the digestive tract, particularly the stomach and intestines. It's most commonly viral. A child with a simple gastro infection will have diarrhoea, which may be accompanied by nausea, vomiting and tummy cramps.

Of course, gastro is not the only cause of vomiting and/or diarrhoea in kids. There are many causes, some of which are serious. In this section, we are going to talk about simple gastro. Seasoned carers can spot gastro a mile off, and if it has gone through your child's day-care centre or class at school (and then the whole family), you can often recognise it.

Prevention

Viral gastro can be highly contagious. It can spread through a class or family like wildfire. Is it possible to prevent the spread? Yes, there are things that you can do to help. Mind you, if your child does *Exorcist*-style vomiting all over you, chances are you are going to end up with gastro too.

My husband and I were away with a group of friends when the kids were little, all sharing a house together. One of the toddlers started vomiting and had diarrhoea. I immediately went into action mode, making sure every surface the little boy touched was cleaned and the other kids were kept away. After a long night, he was better in the morning and eating some toast, but his bleary-eyed mum was not thinking and ate his crusts. Eight hours later he was feeling great, but his poor mum was laid out flat with crazy vomiting and diarrhoea. Not fun.

There are many different viruses and bacteria that cause gastro, rotavirus being a particularly nasty one. Fortunately, young babies can be immunised. Since the introduction of the rotavirus vaccine in Australia, there has been around a 70 per cent reduction in rotavirus hospitalisations in children younger than five years of age. Good news!

The essential things you can do to help prevent the spread of gastro are:

+ **Wash your hands**
  Washing your hands is the simplest yet most effective way to curb the spread of gastro. A quick flick under the tap doesn't cut it. You need to wash with warm water and soap for a minimum of 30 seconds every time you are in contact with the sick person, before eating or preparing food and especially after cleaning up diarrhoea or vomit. Soap and water should be your first choice, but hand sanitiser is fine too.

+ **Don't share food or toys**
  For parents, the crusts off our kids' toast or their leftovers are a bona fide food group. But here's the rub: you will catch whatever they have. The same goes for kisses. When your child

has gastro, stick to cuddles and save the kisses for when they are better. Cleaning toys and bathrooms every day will also keep the risk of contamination down.

+ **Keep your child at home**

This is *so incredibly important*. You need to be in self-imposed isolation if gastro has hit your house. No day-care centre or school (or workplace if you are sick yourself) until the child has been symptom-free for **24 hours**. That's right — they are still contagious until the symptoms have been gone for 24 hours.

Recognition

If your child has a simple viral gastro, the usual symptoms may include:

+ Intermittent, crampy tummy pain, often worse just before a vomit
+ Nausea and vomiting that usually last for one to two days
+ Diarrhoea that may last for a week

It is very important that you seek prompt medical help if your child has the following:

+ Severe abdominal (tummy) pain
+ Diarrhoea for more than 10 days
+ Blood in their poo or vomit
+ The *look* of being very sick (see **The Generally Unwell Child**, pages 182–185)
+ Bilious vomit (bile is the colour of green grass)
+ Vomiting but no diarrhoea
+ Vomiting and/or diarrhoea in a baby less than six months old
+ Projectile vomiting

And of course, see your GP if your child is showing any other symptoms that concern you.

Response

When a child has gastro, she may be more lethargic than usual but still alert and interested, and she may have a mild fever. All babies under six months old with gastro need to see a doctor straight away. But if your child is older than six months, the important thing to remember is that there is no specific treatment. It is all about making sure more fluids go in than come out, so your child doesn't become dehydrated. It is NOT recommended to give medication to stop the diarrhoea.

However, a child with gastro needs more than just water. If your child is breastfed, breast milk is the best fluid for her. Non-breastfed babies and children need an electrolyte solution to replace the salts and sugars they are losing through vomiting and diarrhoea. The fluid of choice is an oral rehydration solution such as Gastrolyte, Hydralyte or Pedialyte, all of which come in different forms and flavours, including icy poles, which makes them tantalising for children. Sports drinks are not recommended. If an oral rehydration solution is not available, you can try one part lemonade or apple juice to four parts water. The lemonade or apple juice must be diluted. Remember, though, that breast milk or oral hydration solution is best.

When you're giving fluids to a child with gastro, you will find that if you give her a large amount of fluid she will probably bring it straight back up again. The fluid is much more likely to stay down if you give her small amounts frequently. Around 15 millilitres every 15 minutes (about 60 millilitres per hour) for a child under five is a good guide. This should be increased to around 100 millilitres per hour in a child over five. Use any device you can to get the fluid into her — a syringe, cup, spoon or whatever she is willing to take the fluid from. Syringes can be quite useful for squirting small amounts in frequently. Be patient, stay calm and don't give up.

The research also shows that it helps recovery if you reintroduce normal foods into your child's diet as soon as the vomiting stops (or within 24 hours), even if she still has diarrhoea. Give her what she feels like eating — within reason, of course! Formula-fed babies should be given full-strength, not diluted, formula.

So, what do you do if your child is throwing a tantrum and refusing to drink? For starters, if she has the energy to protest this is a good sign. It is the thirsty, lethargic child who worries me more. Don't withhold fluids if your child is thirsty, just frequently offer her

small amounts. You need to be alert for signs of dehydration.
A dehydrated child needs medical attention.

Signs of dehydration include:

+ Dry mouth or lips
+ Pale or abnormal colour
+ No tears when crying
+ Reduced reduced urine output
+ Tenting skin (when you pinch the skin and it stays pinched),
  a sign of severe dehydration
+ Cold feet and hands
+ Lethargy and/or floppiness
+ A sunken fontanelle in infants
+ Unsettled behaviour

As I have said earlier, Trust your instincts. If you are concerned about
your child for any reason, seek medical help straight away.

SUMMARY

+ The expected symptoms of gastroenteritis are diarrhoea,
  crampy, intermittent tummy pain, nausea and vomiting.
+ Wash your hands with soap and water to prevent the
  gastro from spreading.
+ Babies under six months must be seen by a doctor
+ Breast milk or oral rehydration solutions are the best
  fluids to give.
+ Give small amounts of rehydration fluid frequently
+ Resume normal foods as soon as the vomiting stops
  (or within 24 hours).
+ Seek medical help if you are concerned, or your child
  looks very unwell or is not getting better.

Family members struck by gastro 'were dropping like flies'

On our annual Easter holiday, we bring everyone. The grandparents, grandkids, children and partners all come together to celebrate and have a much-needed break. This leaves no time for distractions, let alone illness.

On one particular Easter holiday, I woke up one morning feeling very unwell. At first I wasn't sure why, although soon after I woke, I heard my young nephew vomiting next door. In the next few hours, my brother-in-law became sick. By the next day, family members were dropping like flies.

After everyone claimed to be feeling better, we went to the beach for a picnic lunch. Sure enough, people slowly began to leave, all of them feeling quite sick. At the time, we only had one child, and while she was out with her father, she also complained about feeling very unwell. On the way home, she began to vomit all over the car from her car seat. By the end of the holiday, everyone had gastro, and at the time we were very grateful the house had three toilets, three bathrooms and a laundry.

We have since learned how to prevent it from spreading and deal effectively with the symptoms. We now bring the hand sanitiser with us on all family holidays.

Kristin

BREATHING PROBLEMS

Kids with breathing problems are a common sight in the emergency department. It's one of the main reasons why children are admitted to hospital. Breathing problems can affect children any age, and regardless of whether your child is a baby or heading quickly for her teens, it is so important to make sure you know the signs to look for and when to seek medical help. Causes of breathing problems can include diagnosed medical conditions such as asthma, infections from viruses or bacteria, inhaled foreign bodies and poisoning, but these are just a few of many. In fact, to explore every cause of breathing problems in children would require me to write a whole book on this subject alone. Instead, I want to tell you about the signs to look for no matter what the reason might be. Remember, it is the doctor's job to diagnose *what* is wrong; you just need to know *when* to seek help.

I've said this many times throughout this book, but here it is again: *you* know what is normal for your child. When it comes to breathing problems, trust me: you will know if your child is having difficulty breathing. It looks different from normal. For new parents, it can be a shock when they bring their baby home and notice that she breathes much faster than an adult, breathes irregularly (periodic breathing), or is what is known as an obligate nasal breather (they prefer to breathe through their nose). Babies are also diaphragmatic breathers (you'll see their tummies, rather than their chests, move up and down with each breath). Despite all this newness, parents very quickly get to know what is normal for their child.

Why are children at higher risk when it comes to breathing problems?

+ They have airways that are narrow and floppy.
+ Their breathing muscles are less efficient and tire more quickly.
+ Small infants only use their noses to breathe, so if they have lots of snot and mucous, their airways block very easily.

Some signs and symptoms of a child in respiratory distress:

+ **Increased breathing rate**
  As a general guide, normal breathing rates are:

  + Newborn — 40 to 60 times per minute
  + One-year-old — around 30 times per minute
  + Five-year-old — around 20 times per minute

  Of course, this differs between children, but it illustrates how your child's breathing becomes slower and more regulated as she grows. Adults breathe around 12 times per minute.

+ **Sucking in at the ribs and/or tummy (abdominal recession)**
  If your child is in respiratory distress, she may start to suck in between her ribs and at the top of her tummy. In severe cases she can suck in so deeply it looks like her tummy and chest are in a type of see-saw action.

+ **Sucking in at the neck (tracheal tug)**
  The notch between her collarbones may be sucked in. If she is in severe respiratory distress, you may notice this notch is sucked in quite deeply.

+ **Flaring of the nostrils**
  Nasal flaring is more commonly seen in babies and younger children if they are in respiratory distress.

+ **Head bobbing**

   This is a sign of severe respiratory distress, more likely to be
   seen in infants. The baby is using more muscles to assist with
   breathing.

+ **Abnormal breathing sounds**

   You know your child. If she is making breathing noises that
   sound different from normal, particularly if accompanied by
   some of these other signs and symptoms, you need to see a
   doctor.

+ **Cyanosis (mottled skin or blue skin colour)**

   This is a very concerning sign. Cyanosis is caused by a lack of
   oxygen in the blood. No matter what colour skin your child
   has, if she is cyanotic, you will know. Her skin will look different
   from normal. If your child has a dark complexion, look at her
   lips, tongue and nail beds. A cyanotic child needs an ambulance
   urgently.

+ **Inability to feed**

   If your baby is in respiratory distress, she may also have difficulty
   feeding. Because babies are obligate nasal breathers (breathe
   through the nose), if their nose is blocked they find it difficult to
   breathe and feed.

+ **Distress/irritability progressing to drowsiness**

   Lack of oxygen and working hard to breathe can result in
   an irritable and inconsolable child. If her condition worsens,
   she may progress to being lethargic, drowsy and floppy, then
   unconscious.

+ **Coughing/breathlessness**

   A persistent, breathless cough is a concerning sign, especially if
   accompanied by these other signs and symptoms.

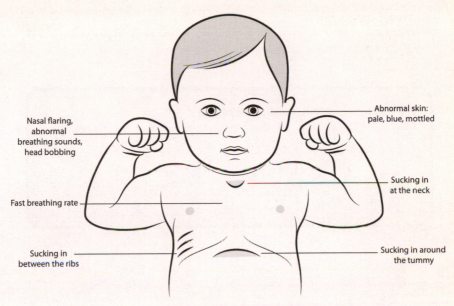

Signs of respiratory distress

A child with respiratory distress needs medical review. Children, especially babies, can get tired very quickly when they are in respiratory distress. If the muscles that are helping them to breathe get too tired, they may cease breathing altogether.

If the distress is mild, you may want to make an appointment with your GP for the same day. If it is moderate you will need to go to the emergency department. Always call 000 for an ambulance if your child is in severe respiratory distress, unconscious, has cyanosed (mottled/grey/blue) skin or is floppy, or if you have difficulty rousing her. Trust your instincts, and keep monitoring your child. Respiratory distress can progress rapidly.

Remember, a blocked nose has a significant impact on a baby who is an obligate nasal breather. If your baby is having difficulty feeding due to a blocked nose, try some saline drops or a saline spray to clear her nose (your pharmacist can recommend one appropriate for your child). A baby can't blow (or pick) her nose, so the saline drops help thin the mucous (snot) and clear it. Babies and children will swallow their mucous, so don't worry if they have a big mucous-y vomit; it is to be expected.

If your child has a chronic respiratory condition such as asthma, always follow her action plan. It is vitally important that action plans are kept up to date and reviewed regularly.

SUMMARY

+ If your child is in respiratory distress she needs a medical review.

+ Know the signs to look for, as discussed earlier in this chapter.

'I felt a rattle in her chest ... I knew something was not right'

When my daughter Hayley was six months old, she came down with a cold, as kids often do. A couple of days into the cold, I could tell she was starting to have some breathing problems. When I held her, I felt a rattle in her chest and she could no longer feed for longer than a few minutes or sleep lying down. I knew something was not right.

At around nine o'clock on the Friday night, she woke up gasping for breath, yet again, and was also running a fever of 39 degrees Celsius, despite having had paracetamol a few hours earlier. My husband and I decided it was time to take her to a hospital.

When we arrived, the nurse gave her more paracetamol and we waited to see a doctor. The first doctor available saw a happy, smiling baby — it was late at night and her mum and dad were paying her lots of attention, what kid wouldn't be happy?! So he told us it was
best to go home and see our GP in the morning.

I did not feel right or happy about this and asked him about the rattle in her chest. He seemed confused but re-examined her. He got me to strip her down, which was when he noticed a rib retraction with her breathing. Realising something could in fact be wrong, he transferred us to the short-stay unit until we could see a paediatrician. Eventually they hooked her up to an oxygen monitor. As soon as she fell asleep, her oxygen levels dropped to 86 per cent. Hayley was immediately admitted into hospital for three days on oxygen. Further tests revealed she had a respiratory virus.

I dread to think what would have happened if we hadn't been able to recognise her symptoms and hadn't asked the doctor to take a second look.

Melanie

FEVER

Fever is very common in children. It's the body's natural response to an invasion by a virus or bacterium (infection). Our bodies are incredibly smart. When we are invaded by a virus or bacterium, our immune system kicks in to fight off the invaders. Part of this response is for the brain to 'reset' our internal thermostat, hence the reason our body temperature rises (fever). Viruses and bacteria don't tend to do well in a hot environment; they would far prefer a nice, ambient, normal body temperature. So a fever is one of our defence mechanisms to kill off the invading pathogens.

Even though fever is a good thing — it's your body behaving naturally — it can make us feel miserable. Kids do tend to cope better than grown-ups, though. The important point to be aware of is that fever is a symptom of an illness. What we want to know is *why* your child has a fever — what is the *cause*?

It is inevitable that your child will end up with a fever at some stage, but we need to remember that our focus should not be on the number on the thermometer. You need to look at your child, just as I talked about in **The Generally Unwell Child** (see pages 182–185). Fever is just a symptom of the infection, NOT the illness.

You can't prevent a fever, nor should you want to. Stopping fevers is about preventing the illness itself. Common-sense approaches like good hand-washing, keeping your child at home when she is sick and covering coughs and sneezes can help limit the spread of illness.

One big concern that parents have is **febrile convulsions** (fever seizures or fits). You can't prevent febrile convulsions and worrying about how high a temperature is doesn't help. A febrile convulsion happens in about three per cent of children and is thought to be more to do with a rapid rise in temperature than how high the temperature gets. A child who has had a rapid spike to 38 degrees Celsius may have a febrile convulsion, whereas she may have a slow climb to 40 degrees Celsius and not have one. Giving anti-fever medications such as paracetamol or ibuprofen will not prevent a febrile convulsion. For more information on febrile convulsions and the first-aid treatment, see **Seizures** (pages 177–180).

Rigors are different from seizures. Sometimes a child with a high temperature may have rigors. So, what are they? You know when you have a fever and you get that feeling of being cold and start to shiver? Your mum might have called it a chill. A rigor is like a severe chill, with lots of shivering and shaking. During a rigor, your child is always alert and conscious. If your child is having rigors with her fever, you need to see a doctor. Remember, we want to find out *why* your child has a fever and a rigor might indicate a more serious illness.

Another question I am often asked is: 'Will a high fever cause my child to get brain damage?' The fever itself will not cause your child to get brain damage. A fever may go as high as 42 degrees Celsius and not do any harm. Remember, a fever means your child's brain has 'reset' her temperature range. It is safe — it is an *internal* limit.

What is *not* safe is **hyperthermia** — the opposite of hypothermia, which is low body temperature resulting from exposure to cold. Hyperthermia is when the external temperature causes body temperature to rise, such as when a child is left in a car on a hot day or a marathon runner gets heat exhaustion. This is very dangerous and can *absolutely* harm the internal organs and even cause death.

Recognition

A normal body temperature is around 36.5 to 37.5 degrees Celsius. Of course, this varies between individuals, particularly newborns. Newborns can't regulate their temperature like older children and adults. If your newborn has an infection, she might not have a fever. She may actually have a low or normal temperature. So you need to make sure you are looking out for the other signs and symptoms a newborn might show (see **The Generally Unwell Child,** pages 182–185).

A fever is generally classified as a temperature over 38 degrees Celsius. The most accurate way to measure your child's temperature is with a digital underarm thermometer. Oral thermometers should only be used on older children, and ear thermometers can give inaccurate readings in small children. The technology is constantly developing, but current research shows the most cost-effective and accurate measurement of temperature at home is an underarm digital thermometer.

When you use an underarm thermometer, make sure you don't have any of your child's clothing caught between the tip of the thermometer and her skin, as this will affect the reading. Hold it in place firmly until it gives the final reading, usually indicated by a beeping sound.

To be honest, the majority of parents and carers of kids will know if their child has a fever simply by touching them. The best place to feel her is not on her forehead, but on her torso (chest/tummy area). Simply place your hand on her chest/tummy area; you will know if she has a fever. One of my colleagues remembers her mum saying to her 'I could cook an egg on you!' when she had a fever as a child, and it's true, a child with a fever does feel hot!

If your baby is under three months of age and her temperature is over 38 degrees Celsius, she needs medical review. These little ones have an immature immune system and definitely need to be seen by a doctor promptly if they have a fever. The same applies to children with a chronic illness. Your doctor should give you a specific plan of what to do if your child has a fever.

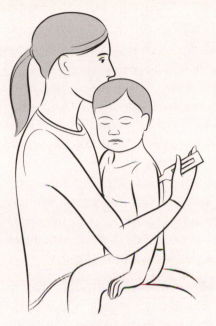

Using an underarm thermometer

A child with a fever may be miserable, or may be happily playing. There are some common signs that you may notice if your child has a fever:

+ She is lethargic but still interested.
+ She is miserable but still consolable.
+ She has normal skin colour, or is slightly pale or flushed.
+ She is sleeping more but wakes easily.
+ She is still drinking well and has good wet nappies (is passing urine normally).

Often carers will describe the child as 'a bit off, but okay'.

These are the expected signs and symptoms of a mild illness. Not all children with a fever need to see a doctor. As I said earlier, look at your child as a whole. She may have a cold but is still drinking well and weeing regularly. You may not be too worried, but make an appointment with your GP if you become at all concerned. Remember, trust your instincts. Like I always say: if you are worried about your child for any reason, you should ALWAYS seek medical help.

If your child shows the following signs and symptoms, more urgent medical help may be needed:

+ She is lethargic and uninterested in her surroundings.
+ She is distressed and inconsolable.
+ Symptoms are getting worse instead of better.
+ She has abnormal-looking skin; it might be mottled, blue or grey, or a rash might be present.
+ The illness has lasted more than five days.
+ She is shaking involuntarily (rigors).
+ She is not tolerating feeds or refusing feeds.
+ She is taking less than half her normal feeds.
+ She isn't waking for feeds (especially important for babies).
+ She isn't weeing frequently (fewer wet nappies in babies).
+ You are concerned for any other reason.

As mentioned in **The Generally Unwell Child**, my two girls had a rather nasty bacterial throat infection a few years ago. My younger daughter had a temperature of just over 40 degrees Celsius. She was sitting up, drinking, asking for icy poles and watching *Sesame Street* on TV. My older child, who had a lower temperature of just over 38 degrees Celsius, was by contrast very sleepy, had not passed urine all day and could barely lift her head off the pillow. I took her to the hospital. The other one only needed to see the GP. This is a perfect illustration of why it's not necessarily just about the number that appears on the thermometer; it's also about knowing your child and recognising when she is not her usual self.

Response

According to the experts at the Royal Children's Hospital Melbourne, there is no point in using pain relief for fever except to help make your child comfortable (see **Resources**, pages 233–239 for further reading on fevers in children). Often parents and carers expect paracetamol or ibuprofen to reduce a child's fever to a normal temperature. Giving medication, however, may not reduce your child's fever; it may simply make her feel a bit better. You still need to watch for other symptoms such as lethargy (tiredness and floppiness), refusing to drink, fewer wet nappies than usual (not passing urine as much), a rash or any behaviour that causes you concern.

Encourage your child to drink; breast milk, water and rehydration fluids such as Gastrolyte, Pedialyte and Hydralyte are all good choices. Watch your child closely, and if you are giving pain relief for comfort, remember to follow dosage directions on the label. Again, it is not about watching the number, it is about looking at your child as a whole.

To help your child feel better, you can remove her excess clothing. Just light clothing should be adequate. No need to completely strip her down, and do not put her in a cold bath. It is not recommended to do tepid sponging or try to cool her by direct airflow, such as a fan. A cool face washer on the forehead can assist with comfort — if your child lets you use it!

Remember to always trust your instincts. You know your child best. Know the signs to look for, and if you are concerned for any reason, seek medical help.

SUMMARY

+ Fever is a temperature above 38 degrees Celsius.
+ It is the body's natural response to infection.
+ If your child is miserable, give paracetamol or ibuprofen for comfort only.
+ Seek prompt medical help if your baby is younger than three months old.
+ Seek medical help if you are concerned your child's illness is getting worse — fewer wet nappies than usual, not wanting to feed or drink, she is miserable or lethargic, there is a rash, or you are worried for any other reason.

'I was struggling to get him to stay awake ... let alone feed'

Our son Charlie was born four weeks ago. Even when he was in my tummy, he didn't move or kick that much, especially compared with his very active older sister. After he was born he didn't cry that much at all, and slept very well for a newborn. An easy and lucky start for us! We came home from the hospital after five days.

When we got home, Charlie felt very warm to the touch and was extra-sleepy the next day, but it was hot and so everyone thought he was just really 'chilled out' and different from our very alert firstborn. However, on the following day, I was sure something wasn't quite right when he hadn't woken up for a feed in quite some time. I was struggling to get him to stay awake even for very short periods, let alone feed. I took his temperature under his arm with a good thermometer and found that he had a fever.

Because Charlie was small, lethargic and under three months old, I knew it was best to take him to the hospital. When we got there, he had to have several tests and treatments. It was upsetting seeing him cry a lot and I worried that something could be wrong with him. Reminding ourselves that it was all to keep him well and safe helped us get through it. The doctors and nurses were clearly taking the best care of him, even though some of the procedures were pretty awful.

Charlie continued to improve throughout his stay and came home a well and happy little baby. I am very glad we were able to recognise that something was wrong and remain calm throughout the experience, even though it was pretty scary!

Emily

Our newborn caught our virus

When our twin boys were two weeks old, my husband and I came down with an awful virus. My hubby was vomiting and had aches and shakes and a scratchy throat. While I didn't have any vomiting, I had the most awful sore throat I had ever had — it hurt to breathe. We were both coughing a lot.

A few days in, when I was feeling particularly bad, I noticed one of my twins wasn't feeding as well as normal. His hands felt really warm, and overall he was much warmer than his brother. We checked his temperature with a digital thermometer but it kept giving us different readings. I thought maybe I had too many blankets on him, so I put him back to sleep with fewer layers and hoped for the best. I thought maybe I was being paranoid and hoped that breastfeeding was protecting my tiny babies from the virus I had.

At the next feed, my little boy was still feeling warm and a thermometer showed his temperature was 38 while his brother's was only 37. It was late, and my husband and I both felt so awful and exhausted. We also had four other kids asleep in bed. But I know a temperature in a newborn is always a concern, so we called my sister in to babysit and, wearing masks so we wouldn't spread our virus, dragged ourselves to the hospital.

It seemed logical that our son had the same virus as we did, as I had been coughing around him. But the doctors decided we couldn't just assume that and miss something more sinister, so they did all the invasive tests including a lumbar puncture and put him on antibiotics and fluids.

We found out a couple of days later that he had Influenza A. He recovered quite well, and fortunately his brother managed to avoid it (I don't think I could have coped with another three nights sleeping on a hospital bench!). We all took about three weeks to fully recover.

Kristin

PART 5

TAKING CARE OF THE EVERYDAY

HOME SAFETY

Before I had kids, I had never given a thought to child safety in our home. Yes, when kids visited me I quickly put anything I didn't want destroyed above child height, but that was the extent of my brief with home safety. Working at a children's hospital is entirely different. For nurses, the safety of our little patients is paramount. Bed rails are always up, medicines are kept in the locked medication room and the kids are under constant surveillance. So, when my first little bundle of joy became mobile, I needed to address home safety very quickly.

If I were to tell you everything you need to know about home safety, I'd need to write another book. There is a mass of information available, some of which I have listed for you in **Resources** (see pages 233–239). Make the time to take a look at this. Remember, prevention is better than cure. We can't eliminate risk, but we can certainly reduce it. Many of us suffer from the ostrich effect — we either don't want to think about what it would be like if an accident happened to us or to our children, or we simply don't think it could happen to *us*. When I hear those words, they frustrate and sadden me.

The best way to tackle home safety is simply to walk from room to room in your house. In each room, get down to child height. Crawl around on the floor. What can you see? It's a whole different world down there. Think about it from a kid's point of view. What looks fun to touch? What things are at the perfect head-bumping height? What looks like it should be stuck into another object (think scissors) or have another object stuck into it (think electrical sockets)?

Then think about the steps you need to take to make the room safer. Do you need to move the chair away from the second-storey window so your child doesn't climb onto it and out the window? Do you need to install window restrictors, which limit how far a window can be opened? Many safety websites have checklists that are very handy to have as you go from room to room. Often just telling young children not to do something is not enough. It can actually be like a red rag to a bull. Tell them not to do something and you can bet they'll be onto it pretty soon afterwards.

One good example of this is when my little friend Julia decided that she would try her very hardest to remove the plastic safety plugs from an electrical socket. Luckily, she wasn't able to, and her mother warned her of the consequences of electricity if she were to play with it. Words and threats don't mean much to toddlers; they learn by experience. And experience she did. This resourceful little girl waited until her mum had plugged in the vacuum cleaner and walked away. Julia managed to pull the vacuum cord out and proceeded to stick a bobby pin straight into the electrical socket (which she had probably saved for the occasion). One ambulance ride, a stay in hospital for monitoring and a dressing on her electrical burns later, Julia went home a very lucky girl, hopefully never to touch a socket again. Even if you don't have curious children, put the plastic safety plugs back in the second you finish using the socket. And push them all the way in.

The following is a brief summary, room by room, of the major things you need to be aware of. This is by no means complete, just a start to get you thinking. Sometimes the easiest thing to do is simply to prevent access to an area by installing a child gate. The perfect place for one of these is the entrance to your kitchen. Read on.

Kitchen

Stove/oven	Keep pot and pan handles turned inwards. Does your oven door get hot? Can kids fiddle with the gas knobs?
Alcohol/medicine	Is it out of reach?
Cleaning products	Are they out of reach? Is the cupboard child-proof?
Electrical equipment	Are the cords tucked away or are they hanging off the bench for little hands to grab?
High chairs	Are they manufactured to Australian Standards? Always use the straps.

Laundry

Cleaning products and other chemicals	Are they out of reach or locked away?
Buckets with no lid	These are a drowning risk. Keep lids on or buckets out of reach.

Bathroom

Medicines	Are they out of reach or locked away?
Bath mats	Prevent slips and falls in the bath.
Supervision	Never leave a baby or young child unattended in the bath, even in a safety device such as a bath seat. Just. Don't. Do. It.
Hot water	What temperature is your hot-water system set to? The recommended temperature is 50 degrees Celsius.

Living room/dining room

Blind cords	These are a strangulation hazard, so keep them out of reach or use cord clips.
Furniture	Don't put furniture under windows of any height. Kids will climb up onto the furniture to get to the window. If you can't move the furniture, install window restrictors, which limit how far a window can be opened.

Televisions	Are they secure on the wall or a table? Could your child pull a television onto herself?
Heaters	Can they cause burns? Is there an open flame? Do you have heater guards?
Fireplaces	Do you have fireplace guards?

Bedroom

Blind cords	As for any room, use cord clips or keep cords out of reach.
Baby furniture	Is it manufactured to Australian Standards? Are bookshelves and chests of drawers secured to the wall?
Electrical sockets	Do they have plastic safety plugs in them?

Garage

| Chemicals and paint | Keep them out of reach. Do you really need them? Dispose of unwanted chemicals through your local council's disposal program. |
| Tools | Keep them out of reach. |

Driveway

| Vision | Do you know where your children are? Consider a reversing mirror or camera, particularly if you have an SUV or 4WD. |

Garden

| Play equipment | Is it falling apart and unsafe? Does it need repair? |
| Plants | Are they poisonous? Oleanders, deadly nightshades and angel trumpets are common toxic plants. |

| **Pools and spas** | Are they fenced and/or covered? Have you registered your pool? (See **Resources**, pages 233–239, for details.) Have you emptied the inflatable pool and stored it upright? |

Bedroom:
- Blind cords — use a cord clip or keep them out of reach
- Secure chests of drawers and bookshelves to the wall
- Place plastic safety plugs in electical sockets

Kitchen:
- Keep household chemicals, cleaning products and alcohol out of reach
- Keep pot and pan handles turned in on the stove
- Keep electrical cords tucked away
- Always use the straps on high chairs

Bathroom:
- Set the water heater to 50 degrees Celsius
- Keep medicines and cords from appliances out of reach

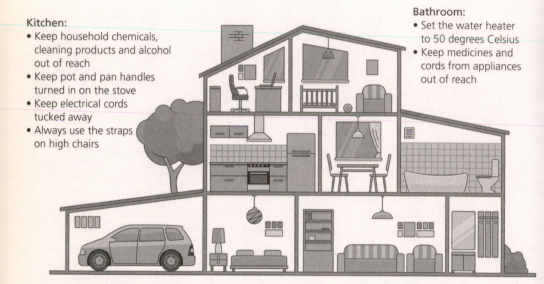

Driveway and garage:
- Do you know where your children are? Consider a reversing mirror or camera, particularly if you have an SUV or 4WD
- Keep paints, poisons and tools out of reach

Living room/dining room:
- Blind cords — use cord clips or keep them out of reach
- Don't put furniture under wndows of any height
- Secure televisions on the wall or a table
- Use heater or fireplace guards

Laundry:
- Keep household chemicals and cleaning products out of reach
- Keep lids on buckets or buckets out of reach

Some safety considerations around the home

EMERGENCY DEPARTMENTS: HOW THEY WORK

Emergency departments (EDs) are hives of activity and controlled chaos. They are often the first experience a child will have of hospital and they can be both a frightening and an exciting place.

Understanding how the ED works is important, because it will take the mystery out of why you have been waiting for hours when last time you were rushed in and seen straight away, or why you have seen three different doctors and four nurses.

First, there are paediatric-specific emergency departments around Australia but most hospitals have what we call mixed EDs where both adults and children are seen. Some hospitals don't have EDs, and particularly in rural areas, the ED may be a clinic staffed by the local nurse practitioner and the area GP.

In an emergency, you need to go to your nearest emergency department.

Some people believe that coming to the ED in an ambulance will get you or your child seen more quickly. This is not true. You will still be triaged and seen immediately if needed, or asked to wait if you or your child's condition does not need urgent treatment.

The most important points to remember if you need the services of an ED are:

+ Emergency departments are for emergencies.
+ In an emergency, go to your nearest emergency department.
+ Sickest kids get seen first.
+ If you are waiting, that's a good thing. It means your child's condition is stable. If your child's condition gets worse while you are waiting, tell the triage nurse immediately.
+ You, as the parent, are part of the team caring for your child — you have a valuable part to play in helping them receive quality healthcare.

What happens in the emergency department?

The emergency department's primary purpose is to provide care to the seriously ill child. For this reason, children with stable or non life threatening conditions often wait for a while before being seen.

When you arrive, a nurse will triage you. Triage is when the emergency department staff establishes how urgently you need to see a doctor. They will assess your child's symptoms and place her in a queue depending on how sick she is.

Waiting is frustrating, especially when it looks like other children are being seen before yours. In the emergency department, this is because those children have an acute (severe or critical) illness.

While you're waiting, the nurses will communicate with you, and if they don't, let them know if you are worried about your child. Most emergency departments will regularly review your child while you wait and the nurses can often give pain and fever relief and first aid, monitor your child's conditions and order tests — common ones include blood tests and X-rays.

When your wait is over, you will be seen by a doctor or nurse practitioner and a plan will be developed. Sometimes plans are simple, and often they involve a period of more waiting to see what might happen. When it comes to caring for children, observation is a form of treatment. They often can't verbalise what they are feeling, so hospital staff need to watch carefully.

Once a diagnosis is made you will be discharged as soon

as possible, with follow-up arrangements if needed. If your child's illness or injury requires hospitalisation, you will be made aware of this as soon as the clinicians decide.

While you are in the emergency department, you can do some things to help the staff keep your child safe:

+ Keep asking what is happening next.
+ Ask for the name/s of the staff caring for you and your child.
+ Ask for pain relief.
+ Make sure your child's identification is checked whenever an intervention occurs.
+ If you are concerned or confused about what is happening, ask to speak to the senior nurse or doctor caring for your child.

The emergency department is not the best primary-care option for your child. Establishing an ongoing relationship with a GP is good for your child and you. A therapeutic relationship can be established and comprehensive holistic care provided. Your GP will refer you to an emergency department if they believe it necessary. Children also learn to trust a familiar GP, and as they grow, they can learn about their own health history.

Kylie Stark

Paediatric Emergency
Department Nurse Manager

FINDING A GOOD GP

Imagine you wanted to build a house. You could hire a concreter to pour the slab, a carpenter to build the frame, a plumber to lay the pipes, an electrician to install the cables, a roofer to lay the tiles and so on. You could tell each of them what was going on, but could you rely on them to talk to each other? What would happen if the roofer wanted to lay the tiles before the frame was up?

To stop yourself from tearing your hair out trying to juggle it all, perhaps you'd decide that a project manager might be valuable. You could speak to them about any issues, they could coordinate all of the trades to ensure all the essential things were done at the right time, and most of all they would have a great overall picture of the project.

A good GP is just like this.

I can't stress enough how important it is to find a good, child-friendly GP. They can save you a lot of worry and unnecessary trips to the emergency department. Once you find a good GP, it is important to stick with them. If you bring your child to see the same doctor on a regular basis, then they will have a really good overall picture of your child's development, as well as knowledge of her medical history. This is important. Your GP is the person who puts all the puzzle pieces together. Your GP's job is to care for your child as a whole and connect the dots when specialists get involved.

Specialists are usually only interested in the body part that they specialise in, so if multiple specialists are involved, the big picture can be missed. A good GP will see that big picture and look after the family accordingly.

The best way to find child-friendly GPs in your area is simply to ask other local mums and dads. Sometimes they might be a little reluctant to share, as a fabulous GP is like finding the pot of gold at the end of the rainbow. But keep pestering and they will hopefully give you the information you need. Another great resource is social media. Ask around in parenting groups and forums where you're sure to find lots of advice freely given, especially on Facebook.

Many people say they need to wait weeks to see their GP but a good practice will have urgent appointments available, especially for children. So yes, you might wait two weeks to see Dr Bloggs for the wart on Junior's big toe that has been there for two years, but they will often squeeze you in for an acute problem, and especially if your child is sick.

SUMMARY

+ A child-friendly GP is essential.
+ Your GP can look after the family as a whole.
+ A GP can put the puzzle pieces together to figure out the bigger picture.
+ Ask other mums and dads local to recommend a GP.

The value of a good family GP

I have been a GP for over 20 years and in that time have looked after countless kids and their families.

It has been an incredible privilege to see kids go from positive pregnancy tests to young adults and in some cases, on to parenthood themselves. We have formed powerful bonds of trust, understanding and respect that can only happen with having known each other for all this time. It's an invaluable asset to have a GP who knows you and your family. We are here to care for you from birth to death. We become a part of the family.

Look around for a GP who suits your style. Work with them and ensure that you share similar goals and expectations. Ask them about how your child and your family can benefit from being in the GP's care. Do they do urgent appointments? What after-hours arrangements do they have? Are they happy to see children? Do they have a child-friendly environment and staff?

Children respond well to being noticed and treated with interest and respect. Everyone wins when you have a happy and cooperative child.

Find yourself a good GP. Treat them well. Work with them and the rewards will be priceless.

Dr M
General practitioner

FIRST-AID KITS & TEACHING CHILDREN ABOUT FIRST AID

FIRST-AID KITS

It is a good idea to have a first-aid kit at home. You can get away with improvising with things you already have around the house, such as tea towels for bleeding, folded-up magazines for splinting, tap water for flushing eyes and so on, but having a well-stocked first-aid kit can certainly be of benefit for treating injuries at home. It's also a good idea to keep one in the car for when you are out and about.

There are some not-so-obvious additions to your first-aid kit that will be useful when it comes to helping your child when she is hurt. The key is distraction. Have a few little toys (noise or bright lights are good!) and books, which only come out when the first-aid kit does. One ex-paramedic I know swears by an app on her phone that features a little monster that repeats what the child says. If the child is crying, the monster starts to cry too. It's an absolutely brilliant way to distract a crying child, but again, reserve these forms of entertainment for first-aid situations, otherwise they will lose their ability to distract.

The other unexpected necessary item is a kitchen timer. Children are more likely to cooperate with your first-aid treatment if they know there is an end point. Set a timer and explain that when the timer goes off, what you are doing will stop.

Here are my other suggestions for a comprehensive, child-friendly family first-aid kit for your home and car:

+ A cold pack — kept in the fridge or freezer for bumps, swelling, bruising
+ Band-Aids or plastic strips in assorted shapes — for bleeding wounds
+ An antiseptic cream of your choice — for wounds
+ A digital underarm thermometer
+ A rescue blanket — to keep an injured person warm
+ Adhesive tape — to keep dressings in place and hold bandages together
+ Eye pads — for eye injuries such as cuts
+ Paper or Styrofoam cups — for eye injuries such as foreign bodies
+ Ampoules of saline — for flushing eyes and cleaning wounds
+ Gloves — to protect yourself
+ Scissors
+ Tweezers
+ Splinter probes — to make removal of splinters easier
+ A light stick — for use in the dark to attract attention, for instance, when camping or bushwalking
+ Wound closure strips — good for holding lacerations together
+ Zip-lock plastic bags — for amputated parts
+ Safety pins — to hold triangular slings in place
+ Assorted bandages
+ A triangular bandage — a sling for arms or for splinting limbs (tie them or use them to apply pressure)
+ Antiseptic wipes
+ Sterile gauze swabs — useful for everything!
+ Non-stick dressing — for grazes and/or minor burns until you get medical help
+ A combine dressing pad — pressure dressing for bleeding
+ Heavyweight bandages — pressure bandages for snake and funnel-web spider bites

+ A resuscitation mask
+ A CPR guide
+ Freezing spray for ticks, e.g. Wartoff
+ Red-coloured hand towel
+ Timer
+ A first-aid guide — could be this book!

Make sure you regularly check the first-aid kits you put together, as some of the contents can expire. Replace the contents as you use them. Don't forget to pack a first-aid kit when you go on holidays too. It is a good idea to separate medicines from the rest of your first-aid kit, as they can expire quickly. All first-aid kits must be kept out of reach of children.

TEACHING CHILDREN ABOUT FIRST AID

As a parent, you can be tempted to coerce your child into being cooperative by telling her something won't hurt, when it actually will. This isn't a good plan, because she will lose trust in you, and if you ever need to do the first-aid treatment again, it will be difficult. Always tell children the truth about what you are doing, or what the doctor needs to do to make them better. If it is going to hurt, explain to them that it will hurt but the pain will stop, and try to quantify it.

A good example is cleaning grazes. It stings. A lot. Rather than telling your child it won't hurt, explain it will sting (or whatever word for pain your child understands), but once it is clean and the Band-Aid is on, the stinging will stop. You might want to use the timer I mentioned earlier. If your child wants to help, let her. In fact, always let a child be involved in her own care. Assigning her a task gives her a sense of control as well as a distraction. Of course, there are certain things that only you or the doctor can do, but even something as simple as getting her to hold a bandage or undo a Band-Aid packet can work wonders.

Children as young as three years old can be taught to call 000, as well as how to roll an adult or another child into the recovery position if that person is in an accident or is very unwell. See **Calling 000** (pages 52–60) for suggestions on finding fun games and apps that teach kids how to call emergency services.

Knowing how to roll an unconscious adult into the recovery position can save a life. Once your child gets to around the age of eight, why not enrol in a first-aid course together? There are some fabulous courses that cater for families who want to learn together.

GIVING MEDICATION
TO CHILDREN

Giving pain relief medication is an important part of first aid and caring for an ill child. Sometimes, though, young children are very clever at making sure more ends up on the floor than in their tummies. Before I outline some 'tricks' I've learned for administering medicine to a child, it is important to stress this: when it comes to medicating your child, the first question to ask yourself is 'Does she really need it?' If your toddler, despite having a fever, is happy, running around, drinking well and weeing regularly (good wet nappies in babies), does she really need that dose of paracetamol? Does she really need antibiotics? If your doctor has prescribed them and explained why antibiotics are needed for a bacterial infection, please give them to your child, and most importantly, **complete the full course**. However, antibiotics DO NOT help a viral infection. So, if your GP tells you your child has a viral infection, don't ask them for a script for antibiotics. It won't help.

There are a few different ways you can give medication to your child — but whichever way you choose, you must be sure you are giving her the correct dose. Always read the dosage instructions on the label and use an accurate measuring device, such as a syringe or medicine cup. If your child takes medicine from a spoon, measure it accurately with a syringe first and then put it on the spoon.

Bribery may work for older children — a new packet of favourite stickers is a good trade-off for a course of antibiotics. For younger kids, pretending to give the medication to a favourite toy, first can help. You can role-play giving medicine to the toy with lots of praise when the toy 'takes' it.

Unfortunately, when it comes to medicine, a zero-tolerance policy needs to be enforced. Explain to your child that there is absolutely no choice: she HAS to have her medicine and there is no way around it. Let her decide as to whether she would like to hold a cup of water or other drink ready to take afterwards, or if she would like to sit on your lap or a chair. Doing this will allow your child to feel like she has some control, but still she must have her medicine. Ultimately, you are in control. You must lead the situation. There can be some negotiation, but not on whether or not she takes it.

There are some very strong-willed kids out there who will keep the medicine tucked in their cheeks and a few minutes later will spit it out, even after Mum or Dad has been convinced it has gone down.

You may be able to mix the medication in a small amount of yoghurt or another soft food, but you should resist mixing it into too much food, since your child must eat the lot to ensure she has received the full dose. A spoonful is a good amount. Don't put the medicine into a bottle of milk either, as your child may not drink the whole bottle. It is very important you also check with your pharmacist before adding the medicine to food or drink — there are many medications that should not be mixed with food (or certain types of food), as it can affect the way the medicines work.

If your child is one of the truly stubborn ones, it is still worth persevering. Be consistent. She will be a lot more upset if she ends up needing to go to hospital when her infection has worsened because she spat out all her antibiotic doses. Enlist the help of another grown-up if you can to help hold your child. (*Hold*, not restrain — she needs to feel safe and secure, not scared.)

Very early on in my nursing career, a senior paediatric nurse, called Nurse Peg, taught me how to give medication to children. It always amazed me how she could get even the most stubborn of toddlers to take the most disgusting medicine without having it spat back at her.

Here is one of the methods Nurse Peg used:

+ Cradle your child in your arms.
+ Tuck your child's lower arm under your arm, hold the other arm with your hand, and stay calm.
+ Tip your child back slightly.
+ Get the syringe in the side of her mouth and squirt in a tiny bit at a time. Eventually, your child should realise that you are serious about this medication stuff and that she should submit to taking it.

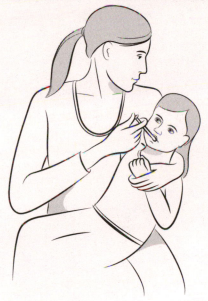

Giving medication to a small child

A good way to get medicine into a baby is to use a syringe, squirt a little bit into the side of her cheek and quickly blow on her face. This causes a reflex that will make her swallow. Repeat until the medicine is all down. Another way is to put a dummy in her mouth then slip the syringe around the side of the dummy and squirt in a little at a time as she is sucking.

Again, always follow the directions and finish the entire course of any medication given. And remember, antibiotics will not help viral infections such as the common cold.

SUMMARY

+ Medicine must be measured accurately with a syringe or medicine cup.

+ Squirt a little at a time down the inside of your child's cheek — this makes it harder to spit out.

+ Check with your pharmacist before mixing medicine with food or drink.

LOOKING AFTER YOURSELF

For parents, hindsight is a wonderful thing. You look back after your baby's tooth has come through and think, 'Aha! That explains the hourly wake-ups and constant grizzling for the past week!' But at the time, you scratched your head, desperately trying to think of a solution to stop the crying/whingeing/clinging/sleeplessness.

Then, just as you think you've got it sorted, your child goes on to the next developmental stage and you are back to feeling like you have no clue. Parenting is a perpetual rollercoaster and you just have to keep moving forward!

Feeling like you're only just keeping your head above water (or, occasionally, like you're drowning in responsibility) is a normal part of parenthood. But you keep at it because you love your child unconditionally. And of course, there are so many good bits too!

To be the best parent you can be for them, however, you also need to look after yourself. It isn't selfish to have some 'me time', or to ask for help. If you keep giving and giving without taking the time to recharge your batteries, you'll eventually fall in a heap, whether it's emotionally, physically or both.

It is amazing what just one hour away from your children will do. Schedule your time off. Organise for your partner/family/friends to look after your child or children for a minimum of one hour at least once a week. I've had many friends who say this is impossible; they don't have time. You can find it. Think laterally. Once the children are in bed, instead of falling back into your normal routine, leave the children with a babysitter or your partner and go to a yoga class, the gym, a friend's house for a glass of wine — anything you'd like to do. And give your partner the opportunity to do the same, with or without you.

If you are a single parent, it can get very tricky to find time for yourself. Consider doing a swap with a friend or another parent in your mothers' group (dads too). Take turns looking after each other's children and schedule it into your diaries so you both have something to look forward to each week. When your batteries are recharged, your whole outlook changes. Something that would have made you explode into a screaming mess when you were exhausted may take on a different perspective. You'll be able to tolerate more and hopefully enjoy your time with the kids more. I can certainly can vouch for that — I am a much better parent when I've had 'me time'. Even that one hour makes a difference. And the children notice it too. My daughter once told me that she likes to exercise. When I asked her why, she replied that she likes it because it makes you feel good, 'like when you come home from exercise, Mummy, smiling and not tired'!

Not only do you need some 'me time' (without feeling guilty), but you also need to ensure your physical health is good. You have a responsibility to your children to ensure you are the healthiest you can be. This includes routine check-ups with your GP, pap smears, prostate checks, breast checks, and cholesterol and skin checks. If you're lacking energy, or you just don't feel right, do something about it. Don't just hope it will go away. What happens if there is an easy answer for the lethargy you have, such as a vitamin D or iron deficiency, and all you need is some supplements?

Make sure you eat well, too. For the first few months after my second daughter was born, I am pretty sure my breakfast and lunch consisted of what my eldest daughter left on her plate. It's a good thing I like crusts.

When you make your children a meal, sit down and eat with them. Often this will mean that they eat more, and it's also a great bonding time between you and the kids. A friend of mine once told me the story of an amazing family who all love and respect each other immensely and, even though the children are now adults, still regularly see one another. She asked the patriarch of the family what the secret was and he said it was very simple. He said that while the kids were growing up, the family made sure that at least three or four nights a week they all ate dinner together and talked about each other's day. He did say that as the children got older this was sometimes quite difficult to organise — what with work, school and sporting commitments — but they always tried their best to make it happen. As a result, those meaningful family dinner conversations have continued. Very wise advice. Use meal times to put fuel into your body as well as your child's, and use the time to have a conversation, no matter how young or old they are.

Be the best parent you can be by ensuring your mind and body are constantly replenished and ready to tackle life's everyday challenges.

The importance of self-care

I can get overwhelmed by the competing demands of my family so it can seem much easier to take my own needs out of the equation. But I find it leaves me exhausted, impatient and resentful. If I get too rundown (or 'blow a gasket' as my husband puts it), the whole family suffers. The briefest breaks from parenting have made a world of difference, even if it's something small like sitting down to eat a decent lunch (instead of just eating my kids' crusts) or taking a 10-minute nap. Taking time for yourself has so many benefits. I love hearing my voice say things other than 'No', 'Don't' or 'Stop it'. I can be my old self again and not an anxious old nag! The inflight emergency instruction to put on your own mask first before helping others is a great analogy for parenthood. Self-care is a very valuable lesson we can pass on to our children, so lead by your own example.

Cath

CONCLUSION

Now that you have reached the end of my book, I hope you are feeling a bit more confident about dealing with an emergency. You might also be mildly panicked at the thought of all the little mishaps that can happen to your child along the bumpy road of growing up, but I encourage you to change your thinking. Instead of feeling overwhelmed by what might go wrong, think about how empowered you are by *knowing what to do*.

This is why I encourage you (and your family) to do a first-aid course. Nothing replaces hands-on experience. Empower yourself with these life-saving skills.

If you are reading this after doing a first-aid course, this book should cement in your brain all the information you learned in the hands-on training for whenever you may need it. On many occasions at the hospital, I have had parents say to me that even though they did a first-aid course they believed they had forgotten all the information they'd learned. Then, at the time of the emergency, they were able to recall what they needed. Refreshing your memory by reading this book every now and then will certainly help with this recall. So will regularly refreshing your skills with another hands-on course. The information in this book is best practice at the time of printing, but bear in mind that the medical world is constantly finding ways to do things better. Make sure you stay up to date.

Another reason to do a face-to-face first-aid course is that most of us are visual and kinaesthetic learners. We learn and retain information by seeing it and practising it ourselves. Yes, it is true that some first-aid courses are dry and boring, and involve written tests and not much hands-on time, but there are also lots out there that make the learning fun and relevant, such as the one we offer at CPR Kids.

Keep reading this book over and over. Make notes in the the back of the book. Dog-ear the pages that are relevant to you so you can flick to them when you need the information in a hurry.

And most importantly, keep up to date with your first-aid knowledge so you will **never** be the parent who says, 'I didn't know what to do.'

Sarah

ACKNOWLEDGEMENTS

To the nurses, doctors, paramedics, allied health, other health, safety and academic professionals who have shared their stories — you have brought this book to life. Thank you for passing on your wise words and experience.

To the parents and carers who have shared their stories — thank you for telling us about these raw moments of your lives. We are privileged to read your words.

My family — my everything. This is for you.

Sally Murray — no words. Just an emoticon ☺ and eternal friendship.

Johanna Roberts — thank you for your illustrations.

Helen, Lu and the team at HarperCollins — thank you for believing a book like mine can have a tangible impact on the community.

The CPR Kids family — thank you for quietly changing lives on a daily basis.

To all the families I have been privileged to care for — thank you for showing me that everyone has a story and encouraging me to be grateful for every day.

And most importantly, the reason I truly love what I do: the kids.

RESOURCES: HEALTH SERVICES AVAILABLE TO MY FAMILY

As I wrote earlier, having a good GP is the cornerstone of family health. But what happens if your GP isn't open? Luckily, there are doctor home-visit services that are available after-hours. The important thing to realise is that this does not replace seeing your GP; it is simply to tide you over until the morning. Good home-visit doctors will send a report to your GP after they have seen you.

Your local maternal and child health centre is also a great resource for non-urgent concerns, particularly around feeding, growth and development.

And, as previously stressed, you need to remember that emergency departments are for emergencies. There is a triage system, and the sickest will always be seen first. For non-acute health issues and mild illnesses, see your GP.

On the following pages is just a small selection of the resources available to help parents. There is so much out there that listing everything would require several books. Details are current at the time of printing; a quick internet search will point you in the right direction if a link fails or you have any trouble finding the resources listed here.

In this section I have tried to list Australia-wide resources, and websites that have links to many other resources on that particular subject.

Just make sure you seek help and advice when you need it. And remember that you don't need to go through any aspect of parenting alone. There is absolutely nothing shameful about asking for help.

FIRST-AID COURSES

CPR Kids — baby and child first-aid classes
www.cprkids.com.au

EMERGENCY ADVICE AND DOCTOR HOME VISITS

These services are available 24 hours a day, seven days a week and are Australia-wide (unless otherwise indicated).

Poisons Information
13 11 26

Emergency Services — police, fire, ambulance
000

National Home Doctor Service
13 SICK

Health Direct Australia
1800 022 222
www.healthdirect.gov.au

Nurse-On-Call (Victoria)
1300 60 60 24

13 HEALTH (Queensland)

SLEEPING AND SETTLING

(See also 'Early Parenting Centres', on opposite page)

Keep up to date on best safe sleeping practices by regularly visiting Red Nose (formerly SIDS and Kids)
www.rednose.com.au/section/safe-sleeping

EARLY PARENTING CENTRES

The following table is provided courtesy of the Raising Children Network, www.raisingchildren.net.au.

State	Organisation	Phone Contact
ACT	Queen Elizabeth II Family Centre	(02) 6207 9977 (Community Health Intake line)
NSW	Karitane	(02) 9794 2300 1300 227 464 (Karitane Careline)
	Tresillian Family Care Centres	(02) 9787 0855 (Sydney callers) 1800 637 357 (regional callers)
NT	The Northern Territory doesn't have parenting centres, but you can call Parentline for support and advice on early parenting issues	1300 301 300
QLD	Ellen Barron Family Centre	(07) 3139 6500
SA	Torrens House	1300 733 606 (Child and Family Health Service)
	Women's and Children's Health Network	(08) 8161 6003
TAS	Parenting Centre North (Launceston)	(03) 6326 6188
	Parenting Centre North West (Burnie)	(03) 6434 6201
	Parenting Centre South (Hobart)	(03) 6233 2700
VIC	O'Connell Family Centre	(03) 8416 7600
	Queen Elizabeth Centre	(03) 9549 2777
	Tweddle Child and Family Services	(03) 9689 1577
WA	Ngala Family Resource Centre	(08) 9368 9368 (Perth callers) 1800 111 546 (regional callers)

HEALTH INFORMATION

National Health Services Directory
www.nhsd.com.au

Immunise Australia Program
www.immunise.health.gov.au

Better Health Channel (Victoria)
www.betterhealth.vic.gov.au

Royal Children's Hospital Melbourne, Kids Health Info
www.rch.org.au/kidsinfo

Sydney Children's Hospitals Network fact sheets
www.schn.health.nsw.gov.au/parents-and-carers/fact-sheets

Australian Dental Association
www.ada.org.au

Emergency+ App
emergencyapp.triplezero.gov.au

Australian Bites and Stings App
www.seqirus.com.au/bites-app

Asthma Australia
www.asthmaaustralia.org.au

Australasian Society of Clinical Immunology and Allergy
www.allergy.org.au

Paediatric Epilepsy Network NSW
www.pennsw.com.au

BREASTFEEDING

Australian Breastfeeding Association
www.breastfeeding.asn.au

CHILD SAFETY

Infant & Nursery Products Association of Australia
(03) 9762 7038
info@inpaa.asn.au
www.babysafety.com.au

Health Insite
A Commonwealth Government site with links to websites that
provide reliable information about child safety
www.healthinsite.gov.au

Product Safety Australia
www.productsafety.gov.au

Home Safety Checklist
www.rch.org.au

Kidsafe Australia
www.kidsafe.com.au

MULTIPLES

Australian Multiple Birth Association
www.amba.org.au

ADOPTIVE PARENTS

Benevolent Society
www.benevolent.org.au

Australian Intercountry Adoption Network
www.aican.org

Adoption & Permanent Care Association of NSW
www.apansw.org.au

Australian Families for Children
An inter-country adoption group that provides some links to useful
sites and resources for all adoptive families
www.australiansadopt.org

SOLE PARENTS

Parents Without Partners
www.pwp-nsw.org.au

Single Mum
www.singlemum.com.au

SAME-SEX PARENTS

Rainbow Families Council
www.therainbownetwork.com.au

GRANDPARENTS

Grandparent and Kinship Carers
www.raisingchildren.net.au/grandparents/grandparents.html

INDIGENOUS HEALTH

Australian Indigenous Health InfoNet
www.healthinfonet.ecu.edu.au

HELP FOR TEENS AND YOUNG PARENTS

Oasis Young Parents Program (Oasis YPP), The Salvation Army
www.salvos.org.au/oasis

Headspace
1800 650 890
www.headspace.org.au

MENTAL HEALTH

Beyondblue
1300 22 4636
www.beyondblue.org.au
Download 'A Guide to Emotional Health and Wellbeing During
Pregnancy and Early Parenthood'
healthyfamilies.beyondblue.org.au/pregnancy-and-new-parents

The Black Dog Institute
(02) 9382 6665
www.blackdoginstitute.org.au

Perinatal Anxiety & Depression Australia (PANDA)
www.panda.org.au

Gidget Foundation
Raising awareness of perinatal anxiety and depression
www.gidgetfoundation.com.au

Post and Ante Natal Depression Support and Information Inc (PANDSI)
www.pandsi.org

Domestic Violence Line
1800 656 463

MensLine Australia
www.mensline.org.au

Parent Link
www.parentlink.act.gov.au

CHILD PROTECTION

Child Abuse Prevention Service
1800 688 009 or (02) 9716 8000
mail@childabuseprevention.com.au
www.childabuseprevention.com.au

National Association for Prevention of Child Abuse and Neglect
(NAPCAN)
(02) 9211 0224
contact@napcan.org.au
www.napcan.org.au

Kids Helpline
A safe interactive place for kids and young people to explore issues
that are important to them
www.kidshelp.com.au

REFERENCES

All references and links are correct at the time of publishing.

PART 1 — BABIES, TODDLERS & CHILDREN

'A Picture of Australia's Children 2012'
Australian Institute of Health and Welfare, 2012
www.aihw.gov.au/publication-detail/?id=10737423343
Sourced January 2017

'Serious Childhood Community Injury in New South Wales 2009–10'
Harris, CE., & Pointer, S.C.
Injury Research and Statistics Series No. 76, Cat. No. INJCAT 152.
Australian Institute of Health and Welfare, Canberra, 2012

Health of Children in Australia: A Snapshot, 2004–05
Australian Bureau of Statistics
www.abs.gov.au/ausstats/abs@.nsf/mf/4829.0.55.001/
Sourced January 2017

Safe Sleeping
Red Nose (formerly SIDS and Kids)
www.rednose.com.au/section/safe-sleeping
Sourced January 2017

Toddlers (1–3 Years)
Raising Children Network
www.raisingchildren.net.au/toddlers/toddlers.html
Sourced January 2017

Centre for Accident Research and Road Safety Queensland
www.carrsq.qut.edu.au

'Child Injury Overview'
Richards, J., & Leeds, M., Kidsafe WA 2012
www.iccwa.org.au/useruploads/files/child_injury_review_and_
consultation.pdf
Sourced January 2017

'Hospitalised Injury in Children and Young People 2011–12'
Pointer, S., Injury Research and Statistics Series No. 91, Cat. No.
INJCAT 167, Australian Institute of Health and Welfare, Canberra,
2014

PART 2 — CPR & CALLING FOR HELP

CALLING 000

How to Call Triple Zero (000)
Australian Government Attorney-General's Department
www.triplezero.gov.au/Pages/HowtocallTripleZero(000).aspx

Ambulance Victoria
www.ambulance.vic.gov.au/Education/Calling-Triple-0.html

PART 3 — FIRST AID FOR COMMON INJURIES & SITUATIONS

ALLERGIC REACTION & ANAPHYLAXIS

Common Myths about Allergy and Asthma Exposed
Australian Society of Clinical Immunology and Allergy
www.allergy.org.au/patients/about-allergy/common-myths-about-
allergy-and-asthma-exposed
Sourced January 2017

How to Introduce Solid Foods to Infants
Australian Society of Clinical Immunology and Allergy
www.allergy.org.au/patients/allergy-prevention/ascia-how-to-introduce-solid-foods-to-infants
Sourced January 2017

ASTHMA

What is Asthma?
Asthma Australia
www.asthmaaustralia.org.au/nsw/about-asthma/what-is-asthma
Sourced January 2017

Diagnosing Asthma
National Asthma Council Australia
www.nationalasthma.org.au/understanding-asthma/diagnosing-asthma
Sourced January 2017

First Aid for Asthma chart
National Asthma Council Australia
www.nationalasthma.org.au/resources/First-Aid-for-Asthma-Chart-Kids.pdf
Sourced January 2017

Acute asthma guideline
Royal Children's Hospital Melbourne, Clinical Practice Guidelines
www.rch.org.au/clinicalguide/guideline_index/asthma_acute/
Sourced January 2017

BITES & STINGS

Is a Human Bite Worse than a Dog Bite?
Commentary by Dr Nick Brown and Andreas Karas
The Naked Scientists, 28 March 2010
www.thenakedscientists.com/HTML/questions/question/2597/
Sourced January 2017

Protecting Children from Dog Bites
Buchanan, E.P., Cesar's Way

www.cesarsway.com/dog-behavior/biting/dogs-children-and-safety
Sourced January 2017

'Removing Bee Stings'
Visscher, P.K., Vetter, R.S., & Camazine, S., *Lancet*, August 1996
www.thelancet.com/journals/lancet/article/PIIS0140-6736(96)01367-
0/fulltext (requires login)
Sourced January 2017

Allergic Reactions to Bites and Stings
Australian Society of Clinical Immunology and Allergy
www.allergy.org.au/patients/insect-allergy-bites-and-stings/allergic-
reactions-to-bites-and-stings
Sourced January 2017

Bee Stings
Mayo Clinic
www.mayoclinic.org/diseases-conditions/bee-stings/manage/ptc-
20251667
Sourced January 2017

Insect Repellents — Guidelines for Safe Use
Royal Children's Hospital Melbourne, Kids Health Info
www.rch.org.au/kidsinfo/fact_sheets/Insect_repellents_guidelines_
for_safe_use/
Sourced January 2017

Insect Bites and Stings
Royal Children's Hospital Melbourne, Kids Health Info
www.rch.org.au/kidsinfo/fact_sheets/insect_bites_and_stings/
Sourced January 2017

Jumping Ants: A Sting Can Kill
Ryan, C., ABC Health and Wellbeing
www.abc.net.au/health/yourstories/stories/2007/11/15/2080163.
htm#d
Sourced January 2017

Envenomation in Australia
Faculty of Medicine, University of Sydney, April 2016
www.sydney.edu.au/medicine/anaesthesia/resources/venom/
Sourced January 2017

Ranking the Pain of Stinging Insects: From 'Caustic' to 'Blinding'
Young, L., Atlas Obscura, June 2016
www.atlasobscura.com/articles/the-colorful-pain-index-of-the-
stinging-ants-bees-and-wasps-around-the-world
Sourced January 2017

Tick Bite Prevention
Australian Government Department of Health
www.health.gov.au/internet/main/publishing.nsf/Content/ohp-tick-
bite-prevention.htm
Sourced January 2017

Tick Allergy
Australian Society of Clinical Immunology and Allergy
www.allergy.org.au/patients/insect-allergy-bites-and-stings/tick-allergy
Sourced January 2017

First Aid for Snake Bites in Australia or New Guinea
Australian Venom Research Unit, University of Melbourne
www.biomedicalsciences.unimelb.edu.au/__data/assets/pdf_
file/0011/2011007/Snakebite_firstaid_ANG_AVRU.pdf
Sourced January 2017

Preventing and Managing Snake Bites
Department of Education, Training and Employment, Queensland,
reviewed September 2013
www.education.qld.gov.au/health/pdfs/healthsafety/snake-bites-
fact-sheet.pdf
Sourced January 2017

Funnel-Web Spiders
Australian Museum, updated October 2016
www.australianmuseum.net.au/funnel-web-spiders-group
Sourced January 2017

I acknowledge the continually updated information from the following websites and encourage frequent visits to keep up to date with current advice:

Better Health Channel (Victoria)
www.betterhealth.vic.gov.au

CSIRO
www.csiro.au

NSW Government Health Fact Sheets
www.health.nsw.gov.au/factsheets

BLEEDING

ANZCOR Guideline 9.1.1 – Principles for the Control of Bleeding for First Aiders
Australian and New Zealand Committee on Resuscitation (ANZCOR)
resus.org.au/wpfb-file/anzcor-guideline-9-1-1-bleeding-jan-16.pdf
Sourced January 2017

Amputation — Traumatic
Updated by Ma, C.B., also reviewed by Zieve, D., & Ogilvie, I.,
Medline Plus, September 2016
www.medlineplus.gov/ency/article/000006.htm
Sourced January 2017

Nosebleeds
Royal Children's Hospital Melbourne, Kids Health Info
www.rch.org.au/kidsinfo/fact_sheets/nosebleeds/
Sourced January 2017

BURNS

'Pediatric Burn Injuries'
Krishnamoorthy, V., Ramaiah, R., & Bhananker, S.M.,
International Journal of Critical Illness & Injury Science 2012
Sep–Dec; 2(3):128–134
www.ncbi.nlm.nih.gov/pmc/articles/PMC3500004/
Sourced January 2017

Burns/Management of Burn Wounds
Royal Children's Hospital Melbourne, Clinical Practice Guidelines
www.rch.org.au/clinicalguide/guideline_index/burns/
Sourced January 2017

Burns Facts
World Health Organization, September 2016
www.who.int/mediacentre/factsheets/fs365/en/
Sourced January 2017

Burns First Aid
Centre for Children's Burns and Trauma Research
www.coolburns.com.au
Sourced January 2017

'Chemical Burns in Children: Aetiology and Prevention'
D'Cruz, R., Pang, T.C., Harvey, J.G., & Holland, A.J.,
Burns 2015 Jun; 41(4):764–769
www.ncbi.nlm.nih.gov/pubmed/25468474
Sourced January 2017

Burns and Electric Shock
Blahd, Jr, W.H., & O'Connor, M., WebMD, updated November 2014
www.webmd.com/first-aid/tc/burns-topic-overview
Sourced January 2017

Sun Protection for Babies and Toddlers
Cancer Council Victoria, September 2016
www.sunsmart.com.au/downloads/resources/info-sheets/sun-
protection-babies-toddlers-info-sheet.pdf
Sourced January 2017

The Battery Controlled
www.thebatterycontrolled.com.au
Sourced January 2017

CHOKING

Children's Injuries
Australian Bureau of Statistics, November 2007
www.abs.gov.au/ausstats/abs@.nsf/
Previousproducts/1301.0Feature%20Article152006
Sourced January 2017

Choking Risks for Toddlers and Young Children
Queensland Department of Health, April 2011
www.health.gov.au/internet/publications/publishing.nsf/Content/
gug-director-toc~gug-foodsafety~gug-foodsafety-choking
Sourced January 2017

ANZCOR Guideline 4 — Airway
Australian and New Zealand Committee on Resuscitation (ANZCOR)
www.resus.org.au/glossary/choking-guideline-4/
Sourced January 2017

Choking FAQs
Australian Resuscitation Council
www.resus.org.au/faq/choking/
Sourced January 2017

DENTAL INJURIES

Patient Education: Mouth and Dental Injuries in Children (Beyond
the Basics)
McTigue, D.J., & Thompson, A., Up to Date, updated April 2016
www.uptodate.com/contents/mouth-and-dental-injuries-in-children-
beyond-the-basics (subscription required)
Sourced January 2017

Evaluation and Management of Dental Injuries in Children
McTigue, D.J., Up to Date, updated August 2016
www.uptodate.com/contents/evaluation-and-management-of-
dental-injuries-in-children (subscription required)
Sourced January 2017

Tooth Injury
Schmitt, B.D., Seattle Children's Hospital, last revised January 2012
www.seattlechildrens.org/medical-conditions/symptom-index/tooth-injury
Sourced January 2017

Teeth — What to Do if a Child Knocks Out Their Adult Front Tooth
Sydney Children's Hospitals Network
www.schn.health.nsw.gov.au/parents-and-carers/fact-sheets/teeth-what-do-if-child-knocks-out-their-adult-front-tooth

DROWNING

Drowning
Kidsafe Victoria
www.kidsafevic.com.au/water-safety
Sourced January 2017

ANZCOR Guideline 9.3.2 — Resuscitation of the Drowning Victim
Australian and New Zealand Committee on Resuscitation (ANZCOR)
www.resus.org.au/guidelines/guideline-9-3-2-march-2014.pdf
Sourced January 2017

Toddler Drowning Prevention
Royal Life Saving Australia
www.royallifesaving.com.au/families/at-home/toddler-drowning-prevention
Sourced January 2017

'Creating a Drowning Chain of Survival'
Szpilman, D., Webber, J., Quan, L., Bierens, J., Morizot-Leite, L., Langendorfer, S.J., Beerman, S., & Løfgren, B.,
Resuscitation 2014 Sep; 85(9):1149–1152
www.ncbi.nlm.nih.gov/pubmed/24911403
Sourced January 2017

'Royal Life Saving National Drowning Report 2016'
www.royallifesaving.com.au/data/assets/pdf_file/0004/18085/RLS_NDR2016_ReportLR.pdf
Sourced January 2017

I acknowledge the continually updated information from the following websites and encourage frequent visits to keep up to date with current advice:

Water Safety Victoria
www.watersafety.vic.gov.au

Surf Life Saving Australia
www.sls.com.au

Kids Alive
www.kidsalive.com.au

Swimming Pool Register, NSW
www.swimmingpoolregister.nsw.gov.au

EYE INJURIES

Acute Eye Injuries in Children
Royal Children's Hospital Melbourne, Clinical Practice Guidelines
www.rch.org.au/clinicalguide/guideline_index/Acute_eye_injuries_in_children/
Sourced January 2017

Children's Eye Injuries: Prevention and Care
Pagan-Duran, B., American Academy of Ophthalmology, March 2016
www.aao.org/eye-health/tips-prevention/injuries-children
Sourced January 2017

'Eye Injuries in Children: The Current Picture'
MacEwen, C.J., Baines, P.S., & Desai, P.,
British Journal of Ophthalmology 1999; 83:933–936
www.bjo.bmj.com/content/83/8/933.full
Sourced January 2017

Eye Play Safe
NSW Agency for Clinical Innovation
www.eyeplaysafe.org.au/project/about.htm
Sourced January 2017

Seasonal Dangers   Summer
Children's Health Queensland Hospital and Health Service
www.childrens.health.qld.gov.au/chq/our-services/queensland-poisons-information-centre/seasonal-dangers/summer
Sourced January 2017

I acknowledge the continually updated information from the following website and encourage frequent visits to keep up to date with current advice:

Better Health Channel (Victoria)
www.betterhealth.vic.gov.au

FOREIGN BODIES
Nasal Foreign Bodies
Guthrie, K., Life in the Fast Lane, 2016
www.lifeinthefastlane.com/nasal-foreign-bodies/
Sourced January 2017

Parent's Kiss to Remove Nasal Foreign Bodies in Children
Koppuravur, M.R., Best Bets — Best Evidence Topics
www.bestbets.org/bets/bet.php?id=1742
Sourced January 2017

Foreign Bodies in the Ear, Nose, and Throat
Heim, S.W., & Maughan, K.L.,
American Family Physician 2007 Oct 15; 76(8):1185–1189
www.aafp.org/afp/2007/1015/p1185.html
Sourced January 2017

'Nasal Foreign Bodies in Children: Kissing it Better'
Taylor, C., Acheson, J., & Coats, T.J.,
Emergency Medicine Journal 2010 Sep 27(9):712–713.
www.ncbi.nlm.nih.gov/pubmed/20581404
Sourced January 2017

'Mother's Kiss for Nasal Foreign Bodies'
Australian Family Physician 2013 May; 42(5):288–289
www.racgp.org.au/afp/2013/may/mothers-kiss/
Sourced January 2017

Royal Children's Hospital Melbourne, Kids Health Info
www.rch.org.au/kidsinfo/
Sourced January 2017

HEAD INJURIES

'Management of Head Injuries in Children'
Conchie, H., S., Fernando, K., & Paul, S.R.
Emergency Nurse 24, 4, 30–40 (July 2016)
journals.rcni.com/doi/abs/10.7748/en.2016.e1578
Sourced January 2017

Minor Head Trauma in Infants and Children: Evaluation
Schutzman, S., Bachur, R.G., Nordli, D.R., & Wiley, J.F., Up to Date,
updated April 2017
www.uptodate.com/contents/minor-head-trauma-in-infants-and-children-evaluation
Sourced 2017

'Fractures and Minor Head Injuries: Minor Injuries in Children II'
Young, S.J., Barnett, L.J., & Oakley, E.A.,
Medical Journal of Australia 2005; 182(12):644–648.

Preventing Head Injuries in Children
Updated by Kaneshiro, N.K., also reviewed by Zieve, D., Medline
Plus, August 2016
www.medlineplus.gov/ency/patientinstructions/000130.htm
Sourced January 2017

I acknowledge the continually updated information from the
following websites and encourage frequent visits to keep up to date
with current advice:

Sydney Children's Hospitals Network fact sheets
www.schn.health.nsw.gov.au/parents-and-carers/fact-sheets

Australasian Resuscitation Council Guidelines
www.resus.org.au

LIMB INJURIES

Skeletal System Anatomy in Children and Toddlers
Poduval, M., Medscape, updated July 2015
www.emedicine.medscape.com/article/1899256-overview
Sourced January 2017

Anatomic Differences: Child vs. Adult
Royal Children's Hospital Melbourne, Orthopaedic Department
www.rch.org.au/fracture-education/anatomy/Anatomic_differences_
child_vs_adult/
Sourced January 2017

'Paediatric Injury Prevention: Epidemiology, History, and
Application'
Gill, A.C, & Kelly, N.R., Up to Date, updated October 2016
www.uptodate.com/contents/overview-of-pediatric-injury-
prevention-epidemiology-history-application (subscription required)
Sourced January 2017

'Bruising, Abrasions and Lacerations: Minor Injuries in Children I'
Young, S.J., Barnett, P.L.J, & Oakley, E.A.
Medical Journal of Australia 2005; 182(11):588–592

'Fractures and Minor Head Injuries: Minor Injuries in Children II'
Young, S.J., Barnett, P.L.J, & Oakley, E.A.,
Medical Journal of Australia 182(12):644–648

General Principles of Fracture Management: Fracture Patterns
and Description in Children
Mathison, D.J., & Agrawal, D., Up to Date, updated June 2015
www.uptodate.com/contents/general-principles-of-fracture-
management-fracture-patterns-and-description-in-children
(subscription required)
Sourced January 2017

SEIZURES

Pediatric First Seizure
Waite, S.R., Medscape, updated November 2016
emedicine.medscape.com/article/1179097-overview
Sourced January 2017

Febrile Convulsions
Royal Children's Hospital Melbourne, Clinical Practice Guidelines
www.rch.org.au/clinicalguide/guideline_index/febrile_convulsion/
Sourced January 2017

Seizures and the Human Brain
Epilepsy Action Australia
www.epilepsy.org.au/about-epilepsy/understanding-epilepsy/
human-brain-seizures
Sourced January 2017

First Aid for Seizures
Paediatric Epilepsy Network NSW
www.pennsw.com.au
Sourced January 2017

Seizures and Epilepsy
Sydney Children's Hospitals Network
www.schn.health.nsw.gov.au/parents-and-carers/fact-sheets/
seizures-and-epilepsy
Sourced January 2017

POISONING

Getting to Know Poisonous Plants
Cox, D., Sustainable Gardening Australia, August 2016
www.sgaonline.org.au/getting-to-know-poisonous-plants/
Sourced November 2016

Eucalyptus Oil and Essential Oils Poisoning
Royal Children's Hospital Melbourne, Clinical Practice Guidelines
www.rch.org.au/clinicalguide/guideline_index/Eucalyptus_oil_and_
essential_oils_poisoning/
Sourced November 2016

Essential Oils: Poisonous when Misused
Soloway, R.A.G., National Capital Poison Center (US)
www.poison.org/articles/2014-jun/essential-oils
Sourced November 2016

Childhood Poisoning in Australia
Cripps, R., & Steel, D., AIHW National Injury Surveillance Unit 2006,
NISU Briefing No. 5, Cat. No. INJCAT 90, Canberra
www.aihw.gov.au/publication-detail/?id=6442467903
Sourced November 2016

Eucalyptus Oil Overdose
Updated by Heller, J.L., also reviewed by Zieve, D., Medline Plus,
August 2016
www.medlineplus.gov/ency/article/002646.htm
Sourced November 2016

NSW Poisons Information Centre, The Children's Hospital at
Westmead
www.poisonsinfo.nsw.gov.au
Sourced November 2016

PART 3 — COMMON ILLNESSES IN BABIES & CHILDREN

THE GENERALLY UNWELL CHILD

'Infants' Symptoms of Illness Assessed by Parents: Impact and
Implications'
Ertman, R.K., Siersma, V., Reventlow, S., & Söderström, M.,
Scandinavian Journal of Primary Health Care 2011 Jun; 29(2):67–74
www.ncbi.nlm.nih.gov/pmc/articles/PMC3347950/
Sourced November 2016

'Acute Respiratory Symptoms and General Illness During the First
Year of Life: A Population-Based Birth Cohort Study'
Von Linstow, M.L., Holst, K.K., Larse, K., Koch, A., Andersen, P.K.,
& Hogh, B.,
Pediatric Pulmonology 2008 Jun; 43(6):584–593

www.ncbi.nlm.nih.gov/pubmed/18435478/ (abstract access only)
Sourced November 2016

'Managing the Unwell Child'
Cootes, N., *London Journal of Primary Care* 2010 Jul; 3(1):19–26
www.ncbi.nlm.nih.gov/pmc/articles/PMC3960691/
Sourced November 2016

'Children and Infants – Recognition of a Sick Baby or Child in the Emergency Department'
Ministry of Health, NSW, June 2011
www1.health.nsw.gov.au/pds/ActivePDSDocuments/PD2011_038.pdf
Sourced November 2016

Red Flags that Signal Serious Illness in Children
Stapleton, F.B., NEJM Journal Watch, March 2010
www.jwatch.org/pa201003310000001/2010/03/31/red-flags-signal-serious-illness-children (subscription required)
Sourced November 2016

Chandler Assessment of the Sick Child
Iliff, J., Life in the Fast Lane
www.lifeinthefastlane.com/chandler-assessment-of-the-sick-child/
Sourced November 2016

'Which Early "Red Flag" Symptoms Identify Children with Meningococcal Disease in Primary Care?'
Haj-Hassan, T.A., Mayon-White, R.T., Ninis, N., Harnden, A., Smith, L.F.P., Perera, R., & Mant, D.C., *British Journal of General Practice* 2011 Mar 1; 61(584):e97–e104 National www.ncbi.nlm.nih.gov/pmc/articles/PMC3047346/
Sourced November 2016

DIARRHOEA, VOMITING & DEHYDRATION

Gastroenteritis
Royal Children's Hospital Melbourne, Clinical Practice Guidelines
www.rch.org.au/clinicalguide/guideline_index/gastroenteritis/
Sourced November 2016
Norovirus Fact Sheet

NSW Government Health, updated January 2012
www.health.nsw.gov.au/Infectious/factsheets/Pages/norovirus.aspx
Sourced November 2016

'Diarrhoea and Vomiting Caused by Gastroenteritis: Diagnosis,
Assessment and Management in Children Younger than 5 Years'
NICE Clinical Guidelines, No. 84, National Collaborating Centre for
Women's and Children's Health (UK), RCOG Press, 2009
www.ncbi.nlm.nih.gov/pubmedhealth/PMH0016577/
Sourced November 2016

Pediatric Gastroenteritis Treatment & Management
Prescilla, R.P., Medscape, May 2016
www.emedicine.medscape.com/article/964131-treatment
Sourced November 2016

Rotavirus Fact Sheet
National Centre for Immunisation Research & Surveillance,
November 2013
www.ncirs.edu.au/assets/provider_resources/fact-sheets/rotavirus-
fact-sheet.pdf
Sourced November 2016

Gastroenteritis in Children
Sydney Children's Hospitals Network
www.schn.health.nsw.gov.au/parents-and-carers/fact-sheets/
Sourced November 2016

BREATHING PROBLEMS

'Nasal obstruction in Neonates and Infants'
Chirico, G., & Beccagutti, F.,
Minerva Pediatrica 2010 Oct; 62(5):499–505
www.ncbi.nlm.nih.gov/pubmed/20940683
Sourced November 2016

'Normal Ranges of Heart Rate and Respiratory Rate in Children from
Birth to 18 years: A Systematic Review of Observational Studies'
Fleming, S., Thompson, M., Stevens, R., Heneghan, C.,
Plüddemann, A., Maconochie, I., Tarassenko, L., & Mant, D.,

Lancet 2011 Mar 19; 377 (9770):1011–1018/
www.ncbi.nlm.nih.gov/pmc/articles/PMC3789232/
Sourced November 2016

FEVER

Temperature Management
Royal Children's Hospital Melbourne, Clinical Practice Guidelines
www.rch.org.au/rchcpg/hospital_clinical_guideline_index/
Temperature_Management/
Sourced January 2017

Fever in Children
Royal Children's Hospital Melbourne, Kids Health Info
www.rch.org.au/kidsinfo
Sourced January 2017

'Body Temperature of Newborns: What is Normal?'
Takayama, J.I., Teng, W., Uyemoto, J., Newman, T.B., & Pantell, R.H.,
Clinical Pediatrics 2000 Sep; 39(9):503–510.
www.ncbi.nlm.nih.gov/pubmed/11005363
Sourced January 2017

Temperature Measurement in Paediatrics
Leduc, D., & Woods, S., Canadian Paediatric Society, updated
October 2015
www.cps.ca/documents/position/temperature-measurement
Sourced January 2017

Myths About Fever
Schmitt, B.D., Seattle Children's Hospital, 2015
www.seattlechildrens.org/medical-conditions/symptom-index/myths-
about-fever/
Sourced January 2017

Fever
Sydney Children's Hospitals Network
www.schn.health.nsw.gov.au/parents-and-carers/fact-sheets/fever
Sourced January 2017

Do Rigors Indicate Serious Bacterial Infection?
Davis, T., Don't Forget the Bubbles, December 2013
www.dontforgetthebubbles.com/do-rigors-indicate-serious-
bacterial-infection/
Sourced January 2017

Fever in Infants and Children: Pathophysiology and Management
Ward, M.A., Up to Date, updated May 2017
www.uptodate.com/contents/fever-in-infants-and-children-
pathophysiology-and-management
Sourced January 2017

Paracetamol and Fever Management
Warwick, C.
Journal of the Royal Society for the Promotion of Health, 2008 Nov;
128(6):320–323
www.ncbi.nlm.nih.gov/pubmed/19058473
Sourced January 2017

PART 4 — TAKING CARE OF THE EVERYDAY

HOME SAFETY

Home Safety Checklist
Royal Children's Hospital Melbourne, Safety Centre
www.rch.org.au/uploadedFiles/Main/Content/safetycentre
Sourced January 2017

I acknowledge the continually updated information from the
following website and encourage frequent visits to keep up to date
with current advice:

Australian Competition and Consumer Commission
www.productsafety.gov.au
Sourced January 2017

FIRST-AID KITS & TEACHING CHILDREN FIRST AID

Talking with Kids About Health: Communicating with Sick Kids
PBS Parents
www.pbs.org/parents/talkingwithkids/health/
Sourced January 2017

Triple Zero Kids' Challenge
Fire and Rescue NSW
kids.triplezero.gov.au
Sourced January 2017

NOTES

INDEX

Please also refer to the First Aid Quick Reference section on colour plates in the centre of the book.